PANIC DISORDER -
THE CHOICE AND
WILLPOWER TO SURVIVE

PANIC DISORDER -
THE CHOICE AND WILLPOWER TO SURVIVE

Written by

SUF SUPIANI

Main Editor: Noorunnisa Ibrahim Kutty
Co-Editor: Dr. Radiah Salim

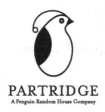

PARTRIDGE
A Penguin Random House Company

To order additional copies of this book, contact
Toll Free 800 101 2657 (Singapore)
Toll Free 1 800 81 7340 (Malaysia)
orders.singapore@partridgepublishing.com

www.partridgepublishing.com/singapore

CONTENTS

FOREWORD

BY MDM HALIMAH YACOB,
SPEAKER OF PARLIAMENT AND MP FOR JURONG GRC

Panic Disorder – The Choice and Will Power to Survive is an account of Sufyan's struggle against Panic Disorder and his gargantuan efforts to overcome his illness. It traces his battle with the illness which was precipitated by not just a lack of support from his previous employers but by their really harsh treatment of employees with mental health issues.

Hence, this book is a useful read for employers too on how to treat their employees well, particularly those who have mental health issues and what they can do to provide better support to them so that they can be effective and contributing employees. Indeed, it is a stark reminder that in many of our workplaces not enough attention is given to maintaining the mental health of employees, when statistics show that globally mental health has become one of the most debilitating illnesses that affects not only individuals but corporations and society at large too.

Sufyan gave useful suggestions and tips to those who are facing mental health problems on how to survive and live with panic disorders. He talks about his own anguish, fears and the emptiness that he often feels and he reminded those suffering this illness on the importance of looking at things in perspective. He also stressed on how support from his family, other caregivers and the hospital had been absolutely crucial in his ongoing battle with the illness.

He described the importance of being occupied in something meaningful, such as animal rescue in his case, so that sufferers can keep their minds occupied and also find meaning in every day existence.

Sufyan's book is special because it is a first-hand account of his own journey as a person with mental health issues. It is a very courageous decision on his part as his book recalled times when he had tried to conceal his illness from other students in a course that he was attending or when he had to go out because of the strong stigma against mental illness. Yet, he decided to come out publicly knowing how important this is to other sufferers.

By writing this book, Sufyan has contributed towards reducing this stigma and also challenged some of the taboos that people have about mental illness. I hope that through him, this book as well as his music album Solitude, people will realise that persons with mental health issues too have talents and can lead meaningful lives given the right support and encouragement.

I hope that one day we will develop into a truly gracious society where people with mental health issues no longer feel that they need to hide for fear of the stigma or discrimination.

INTRODUCTION

My name is Sufyan Adli Supiani and I am a continuous survivor of Panic Disorder. To accept such a diagnosis is never easy, and to declare it? Possibly suicidal. Because Panic Disorder is categorized as a type of mental illness, much stigma is associated with it, as with other mental illnesses. Yet, I write this book – with much trepidation - in the hope that it will eventually help break the vicious cycle that stigma sets off.

My life has not been the same since I first yielded to this condition. I believe, nevertheless, that it is not impossible to get back to who I used to be with time and lots of perseverance.

It all started with me ignoring small stresses in my life, which eventually became too much for me to deal with. Only after undergoing psychotherapy, did I realize that I actually had panic attacks even during my childhood days. The issues I faced were simply left unattended and smoothed over, hidden but not resolved, till I fell deep into a dark dark tunnel of horrors.

This book is the story of my downfall, my rise, another plunge and yet another rise. It has been a long and winding road towards recovery but I am heading there. One huge factor that compels me to hang on are my lifelines - my direct family, close friends, music and the love for cats and dogs.

In a nutshell, two strong words constantly remind me to stay afloat against all odds: "Choice and Willpower". The day my dad accepted me for who I am, embraced me and delivered his single powerful counsel, "Willpower, my son", was the day I decided to name this book "The Choice and Willpower to Survive". I hope in reading this book fellow sufferers will find similar will to survive and others will understand what we go through and be empowered to be lifelines themselves.

My childhood is stained with dark memories, as a result of some incidents that no child should go through. I faced and overcame abuse, trauma and discrimination. Yet I thought I dealt with the stresses very well. It never crossed my mind that my body and mind had limitations. Then at 32, my life broke into pieces like a porcelain jar crashing hard on a concrete floor. Yes, I had experienced my first full-blown panic attack.

I describe in the next chapter the various symptoms of a panic attack. A full-blown attack amounts to experiencing all these symptoms almost all at once. I had the biggest shock of my life. It really felt as if I was going to die anytime.

By seeking early treatment, I learnt that it was not physical death that I was facing but a body and mind shutdown as a result of brain overload.

I understood that my earlier wounds of the heart had never healed. I decided to address them during my psychotherapy sessions. It was not easy delving into these oppressively dark tunnels but through various brain stimulation activities I was able to do so.

Slowly I found ways to manage the illness and was on the road to recovery. Yet, two years later, when I was 34, during a period of extended stress, catastrophe struck again. But this time, it struck with a vengeance. It developed into a disorder that took the form of severe daily anxieties over anything and everything that happened in my life. Be it good or bad news, I suffered severe anxieties, and panic attacks became a daily affair. There were days when these were manageable but many more days when they were not. For three years I underwent and overcame panic attacks. Through the process of therapy after therapy, I acquired more knowledge about my disorder and learnt the art of controlling my body and mind when such attacks happen.

Along the way, however, I also had to deal with depression due to having to fight so hard to survive. The support from my family and friends represented faint twinkles of light while I was in the darkness. I felt as if I was blind. I could not see or grasp any positive vibes. Not because I did not want to be positive. It was simply because I was unwell and had lost control whilst in total darkness.

Have you ever watched the movie entitled "Gravity" starring Sandra Bullock and George Clooney about being lost in space, stuck in a space suit, and having access to a dwindling amount of oxygen? In a nutshell, that was exactly how I felt. Throughout my life, I have always been an optimistic person. I had refused to give up on anything that I did in life. I had fought to hang on no matter how stressful my job was, no matter how messy my childhood was. I am not prone to self-pity.

Yet, to have a lost and floating mind in the darkness with depleted oxygen in my brain was simply not an easy task to deal with.

In the movie *Gravity*, Sandra Bullock would hyperventilate due to lack of oxygen and start to panic. This summarises the situation I was in during a panic attack. I felt like I was trapped in a bubble or a space suit struggling to inhale fresh air.

If you know someone who suffers from panic disorders, or you are a caregiver for one, I do recommend that you watch the movie "Gravity" to understand your loved one better. After years of suffering, I realised that what I needed was gravity. Gravity to stop my mind from floating to places where I could get lost. Often, my gravities are the people who choose to speak personally to me and care for me. They include healthcare officers. Little actions like choosing to listen and talk to me can pull me back to life and back to reality.

I lost the ability to earn a living during those three difficult years of fighting. I had many talents especially singing, my main passion. However, being unwell meant none of my talents could generate an income for me to continue living. My insecurities of living in a cosmopolitan city and the high standard of living aggravated my fears. I plunged deeper into depression feeling hopeless and helpless.

Can you visualise yourself staying at home most of the time for three whole years, afraid of going out unless accompanied by someone, even if it is just to enjoy a breath of fresh air? Afraid of sleeping alone? Not having any monthly income?

The professional guidance of psychotherapists helped me identify the small steps that I could focus on. Most times, I would step out of the house only when I needed to attend my medical appointments. Even so, that took a massive courage and was never easy.

As my condition improved, while still grounded at home, I started to write songs expressing my feelings and thoughts. The few songs that I wrote were enough to produce a full album. It was my dream to record this album one day.

I also recorded many demos of my vocals and published them online as an effort for a positive distraction.

My Demo website:
http://www.reverbnation.com/sufproductions

I recorded demos of my original songs and covers to occupy my time and avoid depression. I purchased Minus One music online to accompany my recorded singing for cover songs. It helped manage my depression because I had a purpose and I enjoyed the process of recording. I created my own sanctuary – a home recording workspace with minimal gadgets – to keep me going. I taught myself through trial and error the intricacies of mixing the music I recorded, and I discovered for myself the basic skills of a sound engineer. This is a challenging tedious process. One day, I hope I will be able to stick to just singing and to have a sound engineer to assist me in that department of fine tuning recordings. I remain strong in the hope that I will be discovered one day by a reliable music label that believes in my talent.

Besides writing this book, my dream was also to record an album of motivational songs to help patients with various mental conditions cope, to encourage them to choose to survive. I dream of them enjoying my music and hanging on to it.

To hang onto something without gravity is a scary feeling. If people would only smile and be happy listening to my music, even if it is only for a moment, my basic goal would be achieved.

My condition improved by the third year with the help of antidepressants. By that time, as a result of making so many efforts to produce song after song, I was ranked number 1 online in representing Singapore for Jazz, Pop and Ballads Genre.

This small success provided me with a sense of hope that my life could get better. The belief starts with me. I told myself that if I chose to believe I could achieve something worthwhile, I would be able to move forward. During the period of recovering, I chose to focus on doing what I could do instead of what I could not do.

I knew I could no longer bring myself to work in a corporate world environment that could worsen my condition.

On the other hand, music has been one of the pillars that I could always lean on.

While the antidepressants worked on my brain and body, deep in my heart, I realised that the major gravity I needed that could keep me on the ground was some success to eliminate all the dark pasts I had previously encountered in life.

Success would help me move forward without relying on and taking too much of other people's time to keep on getting me rooted to the ground.

During my slow, long and winding road of recovery, I was hungry and thirsty to be proactive again in life. Each time my antidepressants worked well on my body, I was optimistic towards the outlook of life. However, when the antidepressants were not working, many times, I felt as if my world was crashing and crushing me. During extreme worst times of confusion, no amount of positive words of encouragements could help - only solitude or the companionship of someone who totally understood my situation. During bad times, there is an urgent need to release all negative thoughts that are in my mind. By talking, I learn to let go.

My mood swings are like a pendulum swinging high from one extreme to another extreme. One moment I am fine and the next moment I am totally impossible – I will cry for no reason and hate myself, feel useless and believe I inconvenience the many people surrounding me who try to help.

Some people do not understand that I am on medication and that my emotions are not completely under my control. When they give up contact with me as a result, it hurts my feelings. There were times where I became aggressive and got agitated very easily. I have now learnt that when all these negative vibes happen, sleep or solitude is the best solution for me.

Along the process of recovering, I have also learnt that anything that we wish to achieve, no matter how small or how big, starts with an option, followed by choices. Once a decision has been made, the work will be done based on the belief system and goals set up in our mind.

In general, when people who have known me in the past hear the news that I have become mentally unwell, their first reaction is disbelief.

This is because, for 13 years, I was the cool and calm guy working in a hectic corporate world environment fulfilling deadlines year after year. Missing a deadline could put my head on the chopping board but I was fine. I withstood choleric behaviours and fine-tuned the art of selective hearing in cases of screaming and frustrated bosses. Working super long hours was not a necessity but a regimental requirement and an expectation in money- driven corporations. I did not possess a degree qualification or even a diploma. With my secondary school qualifications, I earned my living through sheer diligence; I managed to climb the corporate ladder over the 13 years of slavery by trading time for money and I rose from a mere clerk to an executive position. I possessed the right attitude and was very organised, so I got things done.

Nevertheless, my very soul had been shaken by some events from childhood and these would ultimately cause my resistance to unravel.

My stories that will be shared in the upcoming chapters are solely for the purpose of reference in dealing with the underlying issues in order to move forward. For readers who share the same situations, do remember that your life is precious and you can break a vicious cycle with help. When there are too many things on the plate, get help – talk to somebody before any permanent damage is done to your life.

ONE

Understanding Definitions and Symptoms of a Panic Attack

Understanding what we are in for is crucial to accomplish anything, even the simple goals of daily life. Different people have different ways of action with regards to achieving goals. On a daily basis, everybody achieve small goals in one way or another. However, when small goals are constantly perceived to be more important than they really are, there is a danger that small panics will escalate into huge panics.

Panic is like a flame of fire. If it is not controlled, it grows into a huge blaze and managing it becomes a much more complex issue.

The road to recovery begins with understanding the panic situation. For panic disorder conditions, this involves a very deep understanding of the unresolved underlying issues that trigger such attacks.

Due to my complicated childhood and unresolved underlying issues, I developed a melancholic personality. My childhood mind was cluttered with too many adult problems. I observed, understood and was exposed to too many adult problems. The small flame of anger turned into a huge dangerous flame of fire as I grew up because I did not talk about it. I had problems socialising. I was extremely phlegmatic - to the point that I could not even talk when an environment I had anxieties about gave me discomfort.

To forget my troubles, I became obsessed with organising my life. This was initially easy for me because I have been blessed with great organisational skills. Another strength I could draw on was 'good distractions'. Since young, I was always able to distract myself well with the creative mind that God gave me.

Beginning in childhood, I developed a de-cluttering system in my brain. In other words, I would deliberately turn negative vibes into something interesting and positive. The de-cluttering mind-set grew with me and that was how I managed to deal with the executive stress of the corporate world.

For example, at work, I was known to be the guy who could make even a cramped office space cosy and interesting with my creative ideas on decor. My workstation was tiny and I had many files to work with. Nevertheless, I was not negative. In fact, I was able to visualise a beautiful, comfortable workspace. Instead, of cluttering my desk with work items, I chose to feature photos of my beloved pets, landscapes portraits, warm light, and plants on my desk to ease my eyes from the glaring computer screen. I even bought a small fish tank with fighting fish to accompany me while I was working. It was the impossible made possible and interesting. And I was the happiest while working there.

I suppose during my prime days of youth, with a healthy mind, I simply knew how to survive by converting the boring into something fabulous through creative means. In fact, colleagues from other cubicles would visit my workstation just to chill and unwind from stress. I was able to express how happiness should look and feel like and I made into reality the many small dreams I had through my own creativity and hard work.

Unfortunately, cluttering the mind is always easier than de-cluttering it. There is an easy way into the mind, but the way out is not so easy. Cluttering of mind happens when we allow our mind to absorb more information that our brain capacity can withstand. De-cluttering of the mind, however, requires time, effort and most importantly, patience. In panic and anxiety situations, cluttering of fears makes things worse.

It is similar to hoarding situations. It is always easy to amass more physical items than we have space for. Hoarders tend to invest emotions into the items they keep and this makes it difficult to let go of any item. When forced to de-clutter, and the hoarder has to decide what to let go, confusion results. Again, in this scenario, time, effort and patience are the keys to resolving the situation.

In general and normal situations, light panics do occur now and then to everyone and anyone in our daily lives, especially when facing some less than ordinary situations.

For example, many of us have had the following experience – you look for your hand phone in your pocket or handbag and realise it is missing. Your heart races and you experience breathlessness - a temporary panic until you realise that the hand phone is safe, just in another pocket or covered by some other item in the handbag. Then you breathe normally again.

On the other hand, if you really cannot find the hand phone – it really is missing – different people react differently. Some remain calm – they retrace their steps mentally in an attempt to recall where the missing hand phone could be, and look at the options available to them. Others will simply panic even more, and experience a mind block, unless others intervene to calm them and suggest alternative courses of action.

For those who suffer from anxiety disorders, this feeling of panic can be overwhelming in ANY situation – big or small.

I become very flustered about accomplishing small activities or even about dealing with small issues which I used to be able to easily dismiss. When flustered, my mind blocks me from thinking positively and recognising that these issues can actually be solved easily. Matters blow up into epic proportions.

Here are the signs of a potential panic attack. Are these familiar to you?

Heart Racing / Palpitations

Ever received bad news that someone you know or love has just passed away? Ever beheld the lifeless body of a person who used to smile kindly at you? And then, you might have had this surreal moment of shock with your heart racing as you came to a realisation that that person was no longer around to smile at you?

In my case, one of the indications of a panic attack invading my body is when my heart starts to race. It is a bizarre and weird feeling beyond explanation unless personally experienced. If you are still wondering how panic attacks make a person feel, simply imagine yourself trapped in a coffin while you are still alive. Visualise the panic you would experience as you desperately struggle to get out of the coffin and no one can hear or help you. The idea of being buried alive should be able to stir such feelings of fear similar to that of a panic attack.

For first timers, experiencing heart racing may lead you to think that you might be dying, that you are going crazy, that you are going to make a fool of yourself, that you are going to faint and lose control of everything.

Heart racing is a powerful upsetting physical symptom that will terrify you. It is important that you try your best to remain calm. It is important to let your mind take control and tell yourself it is just a panic attack and that you will be ok. Also, tell yourself that it is OK not to be OK.

For caregivers, give the traumatised patient space to breathe. Hold his or her hand and provide positive assurance that everything is going to be fine. A sincere human touch can be powerful as it is part of a love language for the body to identify love and eliminate anger and frustrations. Till today, I will always remember the caregivers who had held my hands during my darkest hours - they simply made a HUGE difference.

I experienced heart racing on my first attack due to enduring anger for over a long period of time. A fast- paced working environment requires peace and quiet to focus. The work environment I worked in had too many negative vibes surrounding me daily. The negative vibes created fears and uncertainties. Seated too close to an unpredictable and choleric management team distracted my focus. I could hear my superiors giving vent to their frustrations. Even arguments about personal matters could be heard despite the supposedly soundproof glass door.

Expectations were extremely high and we were under the radar and closely monitored at all times regarding our work performance.

To survive on that radar, I had to master the skill of ignoring the watchful eyes, thicken my skin and, most importantly, cultivate selective hearing. I felt like I was working under the wing of a dysfunctional family where mummy's and daddy's intense discussions and arguments were involuntarily witnessed. My ears are very sensitive to sound. As a musician, my strength is my hearing and not sight-reading. With great hearing and a creative mind, my mind tends to work too hard when too much information is 'broadcast'. When it became difficult to focus on my work, I was constantly frustrated.

When the low and high-pitched voices got into my head, it would set my heart racing. I would excuse myself from my office cubicle space and make a beeline for the restroom. There, I would sit in the toilet cubicle to breathe and ease off the rancorous sounds. The washroom was an option for me to take flight from the hubbub of office politics. The bathroom was my chamber for refuge.

For a while, this escape and the art of selective hearing provided me with the ability to cope. Unfortunately, being a small fry that had to please both small fish and big fish was just too much. Constantly controlling my anger and allowing it to accumulate beyond my control created so much heart racing and shortness of breath that in the end I succumbed to my first severe panic attack in 2009.

Mind racing

Besides the heart racing, the mind races too. And yes, it races big time. Is your mind consistently bogged down with words like NO, BUT, MIGHT, SHOULD HAVE, COULD NOT HAVE, WHAT IF, WHY?

During the initial stage of anxieties, the above were some words that lingered in my brain longer than it should have. I could not control them and allowed them to linger for too long in my mind. My mind became cluttered and I began having serious doubts about myself. With that, subconsciously, I created a warzone between my own body and my mind, and the root of a panic attack took hold in my mind.

Our minds control our bodies. A healthy body has a healthy mind. They work as a team. These negative words, if allowed to be stored for too long, will create a friendship with a star player called "Worry". Excessive worry will eventually make friends with "Panic". Our brain controls the levels of worries and panics that we face. Nobody can control our minds but ourselves. I have now learnt that I actually have one hundred percent access to the control of these feelings. God has provided me with the access key to make choices. At that time, however, this truth was lost to me.

Nevertheless, it is easier said than done. Prior to my panic disorder, these negative words would linger in my mind daily when the stress level was too much for me to cope. Thinking that my body could last forever, eventually, my mind got disconnected from my body. I never realised that my mind was working faster than my body could cope. I had dealt with screaming bosses, bosses with impossible mood swings, 'loudhailer' bosses and even sleeping, choleric ones, so I believed my body and mind could cope with any kind of boss.

My initial trigger was having to deal with a sleeping supervisor. I had to withstand tantrums when I woke her up for work-related discussions. I was blamed for mistakes I did not commit. Gradually, my spirit and the fire of creativity that made my working life interesting dimmed. I ceased to be the man I used to be.

My body did send my mind a few signals to slow down when I started getting physically ill more often than normal, and required more frequent visits to the doctor. Nevertheless, I ignored these warning signs because the job meant so much to me. After all, it paid my bills and mortgage. I committed long hours to my job. I worked on weekends just to fulfil deadlines. I worked zealously not because I wanted to but because it was the right thing to do. After the 2009 severe panic attack, however, I moved on. I realised it was pointless to work under undue pressure.

I then moved on to a smaller company on 6 October 2010 thinking that I would not need to rush as much; I was hoping for a better working environment.

I remained as dedicated and efficient as I used to be in bigger companies. Nevertheless, I chose to work smart so that I could complete my day job and go home on time. My objective of going home on time was to respect and balance my body and time. In addition, I believed that it was important to have quality time with family and myself.

Unfortunately, my superior equated physical time in the office to commitment. She pressured me to put in as much effort as I did in a bigger company. As a result, those dangerous words started to build up again in my mind. Feeling mentally tortured, my resistance eroded. I began to believe the degrading words and constant belittling of my self-worth.

I began to push myself beyond my tolerance capacity just to keep the job. I knew I could not cope with the volume of responsibilities. Highlighting to my superior did not help as I was given more hurtful sarcastic words. It all came down to the root of all evil, money. The money- driven working environment drove my mind racing faster than normal.

At that time, my mind was obsessed with current dangers alone. I was not able to even think of the possibility of future opportunities.

Now I know that, when in the right frame of mind, there are actually tons of opportunities ahead. Unfortunately, at that time, my mind was too clouded by stress factors. Human behaviours can sometimes be a huge obstacle to deal with, especially when the person causing problems is in power and in control of your rice bowl. The only person who should control you is yourself. You are all that you have got. As I allowed myself to heal the wounds, I realised that inspiration was all around me.

When faced with extremely high stress situations that make you cry in silence, it is important that you put your health and welfare as the utmost priority. I realised that my unhealthy job environment will not be there at my funeral but my loved ones would. In fact, my direct family had always been there, loved and lent me a hand to hang on each time I fell.

Unfortunately, this was all lost to me at that time. And my mind raced to a crash in 2011 thanks to the psychological pressure of working for a boss that did not bark loudly but bit deep with hurtful words. That turned out to be the last chapter of my involvement in corporate politics.

Despite all the triggers of working in an unhealthy environment, I have no regrets. As a matter fact, today, I am able to view all these events of my life as the darker tone of a colourful life. I see that they blend to make my life even more interesting. Life for me has always been eventful. And all that has happened to me - be it great or horrible - are actually huge blessings which I could not recognise previously.

Even today, my mind races at various situations. The difference between then and now is that I am able to control this mind so much better than before. Again, it boils down to choices. I choose the environment I want to be in.

Now, my mind races not because of what has already happened in my life but because I am constantly chasing after dreams. I know where I want to be and I keep doing anything and everything I can just to realise my potential, but this leads to its own stresses.

Sleep disturbance

In a healthy state of body and mind, a good sleep is essential and part of achieving peace. Sufficient sleep brings peace to the body and peace to your mind. Even a power nap can be the means to restart the day again. Have you ever worked so hard on the weekdays and then fall into a deep slumber on a Saturday afternoon? That rest would have been so necessary to be rejuvenated again. Where being able to sleep is no longer normal, where your body cannot rest when it is time to rest, having trouble to focus and cope becomes the next step to deal with, in addition to the mind-racing and the constant anxieties. If you are at this stage, talking to someone you trust and love becomes very crucial and important to avoid further signs of uncontrollable panic. Let's face it. Everyone needs rest. There is a limit to everything. Do not allow your work to stop you from resting. If any big fish ever tells you that you need to work long hours without extra pay for the time that you are willing to commit and trade, it is time to leave for home, have a warm shower and rest. Nothing is free in this world especially when it concerns trading extra time for money. The right your body has to recuperation time must never be subject to selfish demands. I gave big fishes too much, forgetting that I was just an anchovy.

Once, I was in rage and very upset for being discriminated as a single; I was told I had no excuse **not** to stay back to work more and was being constantly compared to others. I controlled my anger from telling that person off and what happened to me? I had a panic attack.

If only at that time I had the courage to tell that person off straight to her face and lose the job immediately, perhaps, the anger would not have lingered and affected my daily sleep for such a long period of time that I fell into deep depression. I was so upset that she did not appreciate the fact that I was efficient and able to execute my daily duties in a timely manner. I hated the greed of human beings but was not aware of the consequences of being greedy. The moment sleep disturbance occurred to me, my mind started to ponder and worked harder. I became hungry for solutions to deal with my sleep disturbance and forgot that options to deal with issues that was bothering me were more important as a first step. My mind raced so much faster than before. It raced so fast that I was unable to return to the current state of mind and realities.

I began experiencing restless nights and horrible nightmares each time I closed my eyes. Without depression, it would probably have been easier to forgive if not forget. With depression messing me up, I could not forgive and I could not forget those difficult days.

From the above incident, I learnt that I did not need to understand everything that occurred because sometimes it is not meant to be understood, but to be accepted. Now that I have progressed with my recovery, I see that the crappy incident had to happen so that I could learn how to sleep better and overcome the sleep disturbance. I have also learnt that greedy, self-indulgent people who are unappreciative of the efforts of other people are simply undeserving of respect.

Sleep disturbance means you constantly toss and turn on the bed searching for a comfortable spot to rest. Eyelids flicker because your thoughts just do not take a break. This leads to a possible disruption to normally functioning during the day. Further, as a result of prolonged sleep disturbance, I encountered two episodes of hallucinations at night. First, metallic branches started to spread and grow, filling up my room when I was laying on my bed trying so hard to sleep. In the second episode, I encountered a strange vision of my cat who was in bed with me – she began changing into different patterns, sizes and shapes.

There are certain drugs that can be prescribed by psychiatrists to ease sleep disturbance. Be sure you discuss your issues so that your doctor can correctly evaluate your condition. Each individual situation is unique and different. However, mental health drugs come with a price: side-effects. To date, none of the medications I have tried, including anti-depressants, help with sleep disturbance.

Currently, while unemployed and surviving, I still experience insomnia now and then. To overcome that hurdle, I choose to live an active lifestyle during the day as much as I can to have a better night's sleep. If not, I distract myself by doing more productive activities such as writing, watching a comedy, gardening and focusing on being caregiver to rescued injured animals.

If you suffer from sleep disturbance, list and write down the things you can do and the things you enjoy doing. Something productive and positive action can distract your mind from cluttering information that stay and cannot be translated into useful action. Information regarding any issue that is beyond our control and which does not contribute enlightenment is information that clutter your mind.

Writing is another way to express your emotions, even if you can only write a few words on a piece of paper to manage the mind clutter. When your mind is fully occupied with too many things happening in your life at the same time, or worse, you are feeling lost, little things you do as an action, such as writing, can mean so much and help you open the doors of other opportunities and possibilities. One word may lead to another word and be an icebreaker for you to share and talk about your overwhelming situation with anyone you trust. Somehow, by writing, the information clutter that lingers in your mind will be transferred onto the paper that you write on as a form of expression.

Keep the notes that you write. Talk to someone you are comfortable with, one who can understand the situation you are in, to discuss about the words that describe what bothered you. Even one word may trigger expressions you never thought you could conceive. By expressing these concerns, de-cluttering of the mind commences.

For those who are not comfortable with words, drawing may be a good way to express yourself. That was one of the first therapies introduced to me when I sought help. Do not worry if the drawing is no more than an abstract doodle. It is the heart that is connected to the pencil used for drawing. Patients should keep these drawings and bring it to your psychologist and share your thoughts about the drawing. You would be surprised as to how there is always a story behind every colour you decide, and the shapes and lines that you pour out into a drawing from your heart, even if you may not be aware of it yourself. Art is beautiful and has no boundaries. And who knows, you might even end up being a great artist as a result of this simple route to self-discovery.

Sometimes, many things we cannot control will come together at the same time. With panic disorder, things may seem to be exploding in massive proportions that we feel and think we cannot deal with. But, in reality, if we put our hearts and mind into believing we can deal with situations, indeed we will.

When things get too cluttered, I admit that my mood swings move like a pendulum rather badly. I can get agitated over trivial matters. Even dropping an object, for example a glass that shatters, becomes almost too much for me to handle. My heart can actually sink just at the sound of the broken glass - I would feel that it was I who broke, not the glass. I would feel like crying out loud and would over-react over something that I forgot to do and things that needed time to accomplish. My best friend, who is also my caregiver, makes changes time after time to accommodate anything that would help me feel better. He has been really patient dealing with my inconsistent mood swings.

Sleep disturbance and unrestful sleep is one of the many factors that trigger such impossible behaviour. Apart from finding expression for your fears, in order to sleep well, it is important to make sure the bed we sleep in is clean, neat and tidy, without too many physical items cluttering your sleeping space. Panic Disorder patients already have too many things on their mind to start with. Therefore, fresh clean bed sheets can make a difference. Warm lights and scented lemongrass essential oil aroma can also calm a person and induce sleep.

Prior to my illness, I was already very particular when it came to cleanliness. My mind can visualise the end result of any corner to make it cosy. I love simple Scandinavian designs. Floral and complicated designs of curtains and bed sheet somehow spins my world around. I also have nightmares sleeping on complicated design fabrics. For me, almost white linen with minimal designs are best to ensure a peaceful night's sleep.

Similarly, it is important to understand what your needs are in order to have a better sleep.

Breathlessness, or fast and shallow breathing

One word to summarise the above feelings in a nutshell: "HYPERVENTILATION". An abnormally deep and fast breathing is triggered by severe anxiety. It feels like the world is turning upside down and one is gasping for air. I do have a history of childhood asthma.

Nevertheless, the hyperventilation differs as it involves depression as well - an overwhelming feeling of massive emotional tensions, where it seems like my central nervous system is rebelling against me.

Sometimes, the hyperventilation is followed by muscular spasms, then numbness of the hands and feet. The numbness comes and goes. However, there are times, I get numbness simultaneously with the spasms.

So, what do we do when faced with such pain?

Close your eyes and visualise something that makes you happy to distract you from the pain. If you are unable to visualise, with eyes closed, breathe in through your nose. Hold it for five seconds and exhale through your mouth.

Repeat a few times until your focus moves to your controlled breathing. Listen and be mindful of the sound of your breathing. Listen to the sound of your surroundings as you perform the breathing techniques. Feel the presence of your body from head to toe. Wriggle you toes when your breathing gets better. With eyes still shut, feel the movements of your toes moving. Embrace and feel your own presence, where you acknowledge every limb as God's gift. The new world of quality breathing should just be you and your limbs. No bullies from real life. Start believing in your strengths.

This will be part of the de-cluttering of mind process. When you are sure your breathing has gotten better and that you can feel yourself and your limbs, slowly open your eyes and bring yourself back to the room or environment.

Repeat the above procedure until you feel better.

Do remember that feeling breathless is part of a panic attack and it is simply a temporary process that you undergo. With knowledge, you can avoid adding further panic to a panic attack.

Nausea / Lack of appetite

Yet another problem you may need to deal with in a panic attack is nausea or lack of appetite. All the depression and hyperventilation will somehow make you feel sick to your stomach. That is why it is important to be aware and activate a breathing technique to channel oxygen to your brain.

Again, a panic attack does not necessarily begin with mind racing or difficulty in breathing. It can even start with nausea or lack of appetite. You feel nausea due to the fact that you are tolerating and withstanding a situation for a longer period of time than your body can take.

We all have a limit to tolerance. You may think your capacity for tolerance is huge. However, your body has a different opinion. Your body reacts to your troubles. Most women in their early stage of pregnancy experiencing nausea would have a good idea of this sick feeling. It is not fun and it feels horrible. I have also heard of husbands that experience nausea symptoms when their wives are undergoing the early stage of pregnancy!

All my life, I have consistently had nausea several times a month. I only found out that I have a low red blood cell count when I underwent the army medical check-up during national service. The low red blood cell count is due to Thalassemia Minor. Doctors always brush it off as NORMAL. Nothing to be concerned about. It was just genetic.

I used to get annoyed when doctors brushed off my concerns so blithely. I did not understand which part of nausea was considered normal. How could vomiting and feeling sick be normal? Today, I realise that it was probably linked to my anxiety of unsettled underlying issues. Each time I board a bus or a taxi, the first thing I used to do was to pinch my nose throughout the journey to control my nausea. My motion sickness was horrible. My mum would bring standby plastic bags each time I got into public transport. Travelling was a huge struggle for me and I often ended up vomiting during or at the end of my journeys.

As I matured into adulthood and started working, my motion sickness got better. However, my nausea would be triggered by stress at work. I used to work for long hours.

Even on weekends, I would sneak into the office to get my work done so that Monday would not be so stressful and so that I could cope with the volume of files screaming for attention. During my younger days at work, I did not do the work because I was compelled to but because I felt that it was was my responsibility to get things done from Point A to Point B. I admit that there are some companies I worked for that were worth all those commitments, as the benefits and staff appreciation were generous.

What got me into depression and horrible nausea was when smaller companies who did not offer so much generosity in staff welfare caused me to lose my health. With time and unattended frustrations, I developed agoraphobia whenever I was in the central business district.

Agoraphobia is the feeling of abnormal fear, helplessness and being trapped in an inescapable situation. I would get nauseated and panicky when I had to walk among a throng of people in corporate wear striding along in a rush. The ring of traffic; the tall skyscrapers; the loud corporate discussions about business, money, property, office politics, mortgage, loans, etc – these visual and aural stimulations made me sick and feel like throwing up. Even after leaving the corporate world, when I visited this district to test my tolerance and resistance, I sometimes ended up vomiting due to nausea based on mere memories, both good and bad. I miss dressing up and going to work like everyone else. Mostly, I miss my colleagues and a few great friends that I had made over the years. I liked personal grooming and looking good used to make me feel good. Ever since I left the corporate world, dressing has become casual and simple. No more long-sleeved shirts, business pants, black leather shoes and funky spiky or messy styled hair to spice up my life.

Instead, I tend to sport just shorts and simple t-shirts. With a mental condition, that is more suitable for me. More breathable. If you share the same situation as mine, do note that it is totally fine to lose, and miss, certain things in life. Take it as a process for you to rest after working too hard.

Because of agoraphobia, I can no longer be sandwiched in the CBD kind of crowd. On a positive note, perhaps there are other environments I have yet to explore and the agoraphobia was necessary for me to move on.

Moving on to new environments may not be an easy decision for most people. It takes lots of courage to move on to a completely new environment and realities. Reflecting on the blessings of agoraphobia, I guess 13 years was enough for me. In a way, I get to avoid meeting the larger than life personalities who had once scarred my life.

For survivors and caregivers, it is important to identify panic locations. By identifying these, you can reduce the chances of a panic attack.

Restlessness

Restlessness is part of the package of panic disorder. With medication and feeling sedated, being restless can become worse if you do not figure out an activity to do daily. With panic disorder, achieving smaller goals is crucial.

It is easy to fall into the trap of deep restlessness. However, there you can get up and raise your bar to surviving. Do not allow yourself to remain in bed for more hours than you need.

When consuming highly sedative medications, I tended to have problems sleeping at night and when I finally managed to sleep, I used to sleep very long hours and by the time I woke up, my body would ache everywhere and it felt like my bones were about to crack anytime. As your body clock switches to a different timing, the feeling of misery and your mood for positivity will be greatly affected.

Prior to acceptance of my panic conditions, for many months after losing my job from being ill, my agoraphobia was so bad that I was paranoid about going to places. I had difficulty staying positive.

It was tough not going out. But the home was my comfort zone and I felt safe there. The change of situation and environment that I had to deal with was overwhelming. The confusion of such mixed feelings created restlessness in me. I got paranoid and afraid easily and panicked over trivial matters.

Being restless, I learnt that one way to feel better is to wake up early before the sunrise to shower, have an early breakfast and go for a morning walk. If crowds make you panic, simply step outside or enter your balcony to enjoy the fresh morning air. Do some stretching. Occupy your morning with simple activities. It can be housework for a start, gardening, and reading or even walking your dog if you have one.

God has created morning with a certain freshness unmatched by other times. An early productive day often at least starts a better day if not a good day. We have the choice whether or not to utilise the benefits of morning air and we have the choice to control and improve our days ahead.

I am thankful that prior to having this condition, I knew and had enjoyed the benefits of early morning activities. With the panic disorder condition, I had lost myself for a while in the storm. It was not easy to resume my morning routine. Every morning was a difficult struggle for me to become the person I used to be. It took me two years of fighting the pain to eventually break the vicious cycle of restlessness. Being unemployed made managing restlessness even more challenging. Writing this book is part of my activity not only to help others cope but to avoid feeling too restless myself.

Besides writing, I also play the piano and write songs to avoid jumping into bed for long hours. To me, an unproductive day triggers anxieties.

Jelly-like legs

I develop jelly-like legs during panic attacks. My legs feel so soft and weak that I might fall. To help myself, I bought a foldable walking stick and a wheelchair in case of unexpected emergencies where my legs are simply too weak to stand and walk steadily. I always have the stick in my bag. The purpose of the walking stick is for me to balance myself once I feel confident enough to stand up and walk after the panic attack subsides.

Avoid being in a rush to stand up during or after an attack. Give your body an opportunity to settle down from the catastrophe. Even if you have to sit on a wheelchair, it does not represent weakness or disability. Take note in your mind that the wheelchair works for temporary practical reasons – at least it enables you to move forward, which is better than being frozen to the ground!

The stick also helps you to hang onto something while in pain. Do not be alarmed if your legs feel numb or weak. In your mind, embed the word "temporary" because once you master the skills of de-cluttering your mind, your legs will resume its functions as per normal.

Never be embarrassed to hold a walking stick or sit on a wheelchair. These days you can get funky and well- designed walking sticks which provide you with style in addition to the functionality you need to overcome jelly- like legs.

Dizziness, disorientation and lightheadedness

Feeling dizzy, disoriented and lightheaded can be felt simultaneously before, during or after an attack.

Before a panic attack, you might be in a situation of high level of stress and feeling helpless. The feeling starts when you feel that you have lost a battle you fought for. Especially, when you are running out of ideas for any options or solutions to help yourself. Having a negative environment does not help. When feeling dizzy, move to somewhere quieter for you to have some peace to yourself.

I get dizziness when in crowded places and when performing huge tasks. Good news, bad news, anything and everything that has news huge enough for me to digest lead me to dizziness. It feels like a violent but brief burst of spinning of the head. Getting up from the bed requires me to sit for a few minutes to balance before I can proceed to the bathroom. Most times, I had to sit in the bathroom. Every movement had a reaction of spinning moments.

After losing my home, I had to rent different places. I get dizziness just from the idea of moving. Packing arrangements require attention and aggravate my anxieties. In choosing to survive, these are the setbacks I have had to undergo. Nevertheless, for the sake of surviving, I had no choice but to keep moving and looking for affordable rentals. Wherever I could find a cheaper place to rent, it had to become a temporary place I called home.

Strange blurry vision

When the mind and body becomes haywire, blurry vision is also part of the process. Again, in addition to de- cluttering your mind, simply close your eyes and focus on your breathing and your vision will clear up. If it does not, close your eyes a little longer. Your eyes may be simply exhausted. Just like when seated in an airplane. Turbulence is expected ahead. The first thing you will be advised from the pilot is to fasten your seat belt as a precautionary move for safety. As temporary as it is, so is your blurred vision. Hang on and breathe. Your eyes will recover after a much-needed rest.

Difficulty swallowing

It is probably a good idea not to swallow anything while having a panic attack to avoid choking. Sometimes, the panic attack itself is a choking feeling where you feel that your throat is closing with tightness. The utmost important tip is that, no matter what, you need to focus on your breathing. It is like flying the plane. You are the pilot of your body. During turbulence, your goal is to stabilise the plane. The same goes with your body. Striving for proper breathing is the only way you can stabilise your body. Your focus on breathing will bring more oxygen to the brain to stabilise your body. It is all about generating more oxygen to your brain.

Also, cry if you need to and do not hold back your concerns. You should not feel choked with unresolved issues all by yourself. If the only trustworthy companion you have is a pet, talk to it. Pets are great listeners. Pets listen and they reply not with words but with affection.

I am a hard-core animal lover. I own cats. Even though cats are independent and they sleep a lot, the affections they provide is simply divine. Cats love to hide at cosy corners. As long as you keep their litter tray clean twice a day, and vacuum clean your home and mop once a day, you can have a comfortable home good enough to de- clutter your mind. Over the years, my cats have developed a clean mentality just like me. The cats and I do not feel at ease until the home is as clean as a showroom.

There is also a fragment of obsession in me in keeping my home clean. When I get depressed, my cats lick my tears, and cheer me up. That is something sometimes humans cannot do. I do not mean lick your tears but being there for you always during difficult times. Everybody is busy these days. Therefore, do not rely on people to make you feel better. Rely on yourself and strive to find ways you can help yourself to be better.

Do consult and update your specialist doctor should difficulty in swallowing persist more than normal. A hungry man is an anxious man. We need to be able to eat and provide our body with energy especially for high- anxiety conditions. With food, we can think more clearly and look at the next step of dealing with situations.

Trembling, sweating, shivering

Trembling, sweating and shivering are common manifestations during severe panic attacks. This is because your body works twice as hard while having an attack; too many things are happening to you at the same time. However, the main focus should again be the breathing techniques mentioned earlier. There are times when I tremble out of the blue especially when I am in anger or when I am simply too exhausted physically.

As for trembling, side effects of medical drugs can make one feel more chilly than normal. Have a jacket on standby when you think you are ready to explore the outside world. When I slowly progressed to being able to walk in a non-crowded mall, I found that a jacket was totally necessary to keep me warm. So are warm hot chocolate drinks and some biscuits – these can make a difference and help to ease the trembling and shivering. If you know you tremble easily, take these small steps prior to going out. Also, do not forget the foldable walking stick – you might need it if something triggers your panic or anxiety attack.

Wanting to run

The feeling of wanting run before, during and after severe anxieties episodes normally occurs when the patient has reached his or her climax of perseverance in dealing with the condition.

It is a feeling of extreme helplessness. You may know or not know the reason. The reason may be either controllable or something that we cannot control. There were periods when I encountered high and severe anxieties numerous times every day. The problem is you also get the uneasy feeling that even if you do run, there is no direction to run. I would feel like I was trapped in a bubble and waiting to exhale. I would walk to and fro, searching and searching for answers when I was not even clear of the question. And when someone contributed an advice or comment for help, the help simply made no sense and I could not understand why.

You can recover

Never underestimate the powers of small achievements for every task achieved during times of panic crisis. Small achievements should be considered part of recovery as it involves courage and determination. There are many underlying issues that need to be taken care of step by step in order to achieve peace. Even if the peace is temporary, it is considered an achievement. Sometimes, we get too hard on ourselves with the developments and progress we make to recover. We tend to forget the little achievements that we have accomplished. By nature, we can sometimes be our worst critics. I have been guilty of that myself.

Also, remember that everything happens for a reason. Choosing to be a survivor will lead you to mastering many skills in overcoming obstacles. God does not test you if he does not love you. There is always something to learn from painful experiences.

Once, I read an article about a story of a barber and his customer discussing God while having a haircut.

The barber and his customer

The barber confidently told his customer that he does not believe in "GOD" because too many bad things happened around the world. To avoid arguments, the customer did not comment.

After the haircut, however, the customer walked out and looked out for men with long messy hair and dirty clothing. Once he noticed such a person, the customer returned to the barber and declared that he did not believe in barbers.

The barber was surprised and annoyed. "What madness is this? Haven't I trimmed your hair? Why say you don't believe I exist?" he fumed. The customer replied that there was a man living nearby that needed a haircut but was not receiving any; that was proof barbers did not exist. The barber retorted, "Ah, but barbers DO exist! What happens is that people do not come to me."

The customer then smiled, and noted, "God too does exist. What happens is people do not go to HIM and do not look for HIM!"

In life, when faced with adversities, we tend to ask why. We tend to be more concerned about the opinions of other people rather than understanding what we really need in life in order to achieve happiness. We fail to see our own flaws but we are able to see other people's flaws. Do not be like the barber who assumes that the existence of misery proves that a good God does not exist. Turn to God, and you will discover blessings you never noted existed.

When I had panic conditions, I never understood why I had to suffer so. But as time passes, I am discovering some reasons. I believe now that God was just paving the way for me to receive other blessings that I could only achieve through fighting and overcoming obstacles.

In simple theory, a dog or any other tamed animals gets treats for becoming good at a task. The same goes for the cycle of life. There are hidden blessings everywhere. We simply need to discover it ourselves even if it comes with a package of adversities.

I must say that, if not for my panic condition, my life would not have been that colourful. God adds some sugar, spice and even some dashes of bitterness to our lives to spice them up. Even the Spice Girls sang about the need to "Spice up your life". And at the end of the song, they say "Hold tight".

"Hold Tight" are two very important words - they give us the ability to move forward on whatever roller coaster ride we have to encounter in life. Hold tight to your caregivers, family, doctors, friends or even furry friends. These provide us with many more options than you may initially think are available.

Reflections

The most common symptoms of panic disorder are:

- HeartRacing/Palpitations
- Mind racing

- Sleep disturbance
- Breathlessness, or fast shallow breathing
- Nasea / Lack of appetite
- Restlessness
- Jelly-like legs
- Dizziness, disorientation and light-headedness
- Strange blurry vision
- Difficulty swallowing
- Trembling, Sweating, Shivering

Various coping strategies I use to cope with symptoms include:

- breathingtechniques,
- maintaining a de-cluttered andcleanhome,
- having a routine that is productive and manageable even when you are unemployed for unavoidable reasons; and
- expressing yourself through writing, music or art.
- There are no shortcuts to recovery, but with perseverance, living a normal life is possible.

TWO

Identifying the Underlying Issues

Peeling onions

A cluttered mind is like a piece of onion – over the years, even small, unresolved issues become layers and if we do not make an effort to eliminate them fast, they linger. We need to peel them off consciously. Every onion layer has a different thickness. Similarly, with our unsettled issues. Eventually, the layers will create a huge and chunky onion in your mind, a parasite sucking your brain juice or a cancerous growth that causes everlasting pain. In reality, when there is something physically growing inside our body that is not supposed to be there, we get it removed and done with. Do the same with your mind - peel it while the layers are still fresh.

When I was diagnosed with panic disorder and receiving psychotherapy treatments, I realised that there were so many layers of underlying issues cluttering my mind over the span of my 34 years. These troubles, being buried inside my head, had never been solved. As such, each time I had to face memories of the past, I would become depressed.

With the help of a professional psychologist, my issues were laid on the table and discussed privately. From my therapy sessions, I was also amazed how many options and solutions I had with respect to these issues. I realised I could make a difference by choosing **WHEN** to deal with the underlying issues hidden in my mind. What I should not do however was pretend I could choose **IF** I wanted to deal with them.

Of course, solving underlying issues is not easy. To embrace underlying issues requires commitment and also a willingness to be helped. Nobody can help us if we choose not to share difficult situations and deep issues relating to your past. It will be a journey where you will not be comfortable as it brings you down a memory lane that you have hated and have chosen to forget. The fact is, it is not easy to forget even when we forgive. The incidents remain in the deepest recesses of your mind and must be dealt with, like it or not.

The good thing is you might be amazed that not all the issues you remember will remain laced with the negativity that we perceived. Through the journey, you will discover your strengths you never knew existed. Whatever you perceived as weakness in yourself can sometimes turn out to be a strength that could make a difference to your recovery and better health.

Facing up to underlying issues

Below are some of the many underlying issues I faced. I would like to share them hoping to inspire you with the importance of understanding and speaking up to resolve your underlying issues, whatever they may be.

My underlying issues started even before I was born. There were many external pressures on my parents at the time, and it could be said that I was literally born to save the marriage.

As a child, I possessed a forward-thinking brain and I had a radar that tuned significantly towards adult behaviour.

Being different, my childhood was stained with the vision and memories of how adults behaved badly towards my parents. I didn't like what I saw and I was disturbed. But as a child, I had no authority to voice out my concerns. I simply stood by and watched my parents face depression year after year. Both my parents are survivors of depression - thanks to their strong willpower to move on.

The picture below illustrates faces of concerned, sad and powerless children. Those were the worst days of my parents' lives, as they struggled to survive ordeals. It is written on the faces of my twin sisters who have health issues. We knew there was nothing we could do to protect our parents.

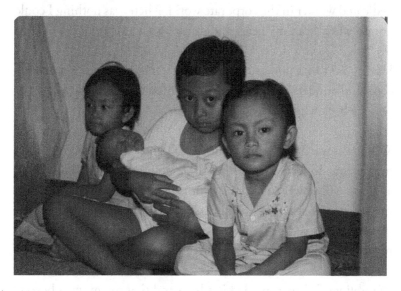

I was a troubled boy who suffered in silence dealing with my childhood issues alone.

Fortunately, GOD gave me a creative mind to distract myself from being too absorbed by adult conduct. When forward thinking is mixed with creativity, visualisation becomes easy. When this is implemented, the results are always gratifying. I am always amazed by colours, lines and shapes that eventually form designs.

Today, I have decided to break that silence.

With that strength, I was able to always make myself comfortable wherever I was and in whatever I did. I am glad that even when I suffered depression, my creativity never left the building. My policy in life is "When planning life, visualise the results in mind". For many years, this policy worked for me. Prior to crashing with panic disorder, I applied it to achieve small and big goals in anything and everything that I did in life. I was a student leader in school and a dedicated worker in the corporate world. There was nothing I could not do when I put my heart and mind into it.

Having said that, life as humans is very fragile. There is a need to constantly understand the importance of not breaking down, but to bounce back when faced with problems yet to be solved.

Willpower was another gift from GOD to me, which I received from my parents. In fact, all my other three siblings are well blessed with a strong will power too. Elder twin is now a make-up artiste while the other two sisters are violinists. I was traumatised with many painful events yet the positive attitude that my parents had towards my upbringing and that of my three siblings helped.

We siblings feel that my dad is a hero and that my mum is beyond being a heroine for her clear and clean heart. She is the Wonder Woman and Superwoman of our lives. She has the "never give up" attitude and that she has passed to her children who are constantly inspired by her willpower.

My mum leads her children by example. While some constantly choose to push responsibilities when it comes to being a caregiver, she takes it in her stride even though she has an adult son who is in need of her attention because of depression. God loves her and has given her the strength to run her own business and to be a caregiver for her husband and all her children all at the same time. Now, in her 50s, she hardly has enough rest and sleep. Yet, she never fails to smile and love. Her love is so sincere that even her business customers call her mum.

Despite all the obstacles, distractions and challenges, my dad invested in music for all his children. I knew that he worked super hard to make ends meet so that we siblings would at least have a skill to hang on in the future. It was not cheap attending music lessons. Dad sacrificed too much for his children. When I had to witness how my parents suffered and how rocky their marriage once became because of constant instigations to break our love nucleus, it wounded me with a burning rage inside me because there was nothing I could do.

Those underlying issues contaminated my mind, as I never really gave vent to those frustrations.

Whatever the reasons of my frustrations, these are no longer important because they are simply the past. By getting help from professionals, one huge layer of onion has been removed from the past.

Do note that getting help from professionals is crucial when peeling off onion layers because the other party is then not involved emotionally. That helps you tackle your wound more effectively.

As mentioned earlier in Chapter 1, I was also born with a blood disorder that was only discovered during my adolescence. My full red blood count is lower than that of a normal male. Perhaps, slightly lower than an average female. I was weak most times. Having to deal with childhood asthma and constant nausea episodes and motion sickness did not help my self-esteem.

When I was a child, Malay boys were meant to play football while Chinese boys played basketball. The mentality was that boys needed to play sports to prove the man in you. My parents were never ashamed that I could not play football because they understood my medical situation. However, as I fell under the Malay boy category, I lived in constant fear and depression when it came to sports lessons in school. I developed anxieties each time I had to go for sports lessons. The peer pressure was unbearable. Often I got teased for being different. I was not the typical Malay boy, so I became a loner.

On the other hand, girls were comfortable sharing with me their thoughts and wanted to be my friends because I was understanding. They sought me for sensible opinions and were not childish. Unfortunately, I perceived this strength negatively. I felt that my mature thinking was too early and rigid. I felt it was weird being more comfortable mingling with the girls compared to the boys. But I had no choice. The girls found me interesting and the boys looked down on me.

My connection with boys was awkward because we had no common interest to talk about. Even if there was, these opportunities were never discovered, as I was not rough enough for the other boys. How could I be rough when the energy that I had daily was so limited? My body was sensitive and allergic to many things. I pinched my nose in public transport each time I boarded the taxi due to my allergy to car deodorisers. I suffered extreme nausea and vomiting triggered by the smell, and also by the constant jerking driving style of taxi drivers. I would also vomit each time I travelled by bus.

These are just little layers of underlying issues I faced throughout my childhood. With time, as I grew up, the layers thickened, leaving painful memories. Some of the girls who wanted to be my friend when I was in primary school are still in touch me. They all have their own families now and I am so proud of them; yet they still remember me as a friend.

The vicious cycle continued even when I was in secondary school where the peer pressures were even tougher for me to deal with mentally.

I was a student leader most of my school days and received many awards for being a great student leader. My efforts were recognised by the school principal and head of departments in appreciation of my strengths. However, at that time, I failed to see them as strengths just because I was not as strong like other boys playing sports. While externally, I was focused on progressing based on the strengths that I had, internally I was focusing on what I did not have rather than accepting what I had.

As normal as I appeared to be, my soul was deeply hurt. I tried not to show my frustrations at being teased all the time.

Apart from a handful of nice boys, most of the others called me "Softy" and "Skinny legs", probably because I never played football and that was a disgrace for a male. It was a male syndrome that I could not understand. Each time I heard loud cheers about scoring a goal at the football field or television matches, I would panic and excuse myself. Deep inside, I was in rage. I simply avoided boys who teased me or were sarcastic to me. Within their clan, they seemed perfect. Perfect physiques and perfect acceptance by their peers.

Boys will be boys. They constantly made fun of my ignorance. They put condoms in my pencil box. I did not know what it was and I dared not ask as that would make me a laughing stock.

To cope, I strove towards becoming a good student leader. I was the class chairman, a drum major of the school military band, and an active librarian promoting books. I was capable in many areas, especially with regards to leadership, despite my low self-esteem during my high school days. Most of my school band members were girls. They joined because of me. I constantly found ways to dignify my strengths, although secretly I saw them as weaknesses because I was not physically strong like them and not playing football but music. I still remember my male classmates strongly suggesting that as a male, I should play football. They even offered to teach me. It was tempting to be what I was not meant to be just to feel accepted. But I could not. My physical tolerance did not permit me to do so.

I was also a jack-of-all-trades when it came to creative work. For music that interested me, I would play; rewind and forward the cassette player just to write down the lyrics. Once, I recorded my voice secretly using my aunt's tape recorder while she was away. During puberty stage, my voice was awkward. I practically croaked like a frog. Someone laughed at me uncontrollably upon hearing my recorded frog voice. That laughter remains vivid in my head. I told myself that one day, when my puberty voice healed, I would be a singer.

And I did. I attended auditions after auditions until I was given the opportunity to appear on television. It was not easy but I did not give up. If not for my dad's investment in skill development for me to overcome my weaknesses with music appreciation knowing that my main strength was creativity and not sports, I would not have achieved so many things in life.

One of my greatest experiences during my adolescent years of singing was representing Singapore and my culture during a cultural exchange program in 1997 as you can see from the date on the bottom right of the photo. An orchestra accompanied my singing and I flew to Japan together with a team of professional musicians. I did not allow anyone to take my dream of singing away.

This was only possible because I managed to convert what was many perceived to be my weakness (including myself) and change it into strength.

My mum, who is my biggest fan, was proud and excited. She sewed the traditional costume below for me. She actually learnt sewing just so that she could sew a costume for her son.

Letting go of the past

Previously, a simple phone with a simple ringtone was viewed with amazement. These days, however, mobile phones are inadequate unless they come with all sorts of apps and the ability to access vast information in addition to the ability to connect a call. Unfortunately, with enhanced technology, the level and quality of stress is also intensified. As internet mobile data is transferred at greater speeds and more memory is need for more usage, so too with our brain. Our brain needs space for more data to enter. It means you need to let go of the unwanted data stored in your brain.

Similarly, while in the not-so-distant past, we were patient with slow internet speeds, high-speed data is no longer a luxury but a necessity.

A natural consequence of living in this new era is that we have executive stress to deal with. Stress management has become a crucial skill that we all need to learn. Without panic disorder, I would not have stopped and paused before deciding to move on. Such is life. We can learn from the adversities of life only if we choose to.

Cultural Exchange Program in Japan 1997

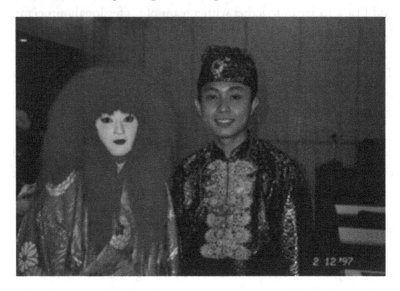

2 12 '97

Reflection

There are actually many complicated underlying issues of mine that have yet to be solved. The ones I share above are the ones that are important for people out there, especially children and youngsters who face similar situations. For those who do, just remember:

- There are some things in life that are beyond our control - the choice is either to give up or move on.
- Do not be afraid of making a fool of yourself in pursuing your strengths just because others see them as weaknesses.
- By accepting who you are, you become free – and freedom is power.

- Be mindful that there is HOPE. You need to believe in yourself more than anyone else can. Never allow anyone to take your dreams away.

Do note that panic disorder is not a weakness. Panic disorder, severe anxieties and depression happen because you have been too strong for too long a period. If it happens to you, take it slow and just breathe.

THREE

Accepting the Diagnosis

To accept news of something you are not prepared for is never easy. Sudden news, good or bad, is normally accompanied by shock and disbelief, while expected news is easier to accept. Nevertheless, whether we are prepared or not prepared to accept the news, something that has happened has become reality, and denying it is futile.

You are not dying, so cheer up

Often, when having a panic attack, I get an uncontrollable feeling that I am going to die. This thought naturally forces itself upon the mind due to the violent roller coaster ride it experiences.

Death can happen anywhere and anytime. Even when seated doing nothing, when the time comes, it happens. There are some people I knew in life who passed on without any illnesses. All of a sudden, that special, chirpy, down- to-earth person is gone. On the other hand, there are some people I know in life who has myriad illnesses and suffering but their time is not yet up – it is up to them to still live a quality life.

The good news is that death is not part of the package in panic attacks. It is an indescribable feeling that only the person who encounters an attack can relate to - the fear that overwhelms you when you feel that you are going to die. Yet, you will not die unless your time is really up and you are meant to die together with the attack, but that is beyond anyone's control.

This is one reason one needs to accept the diagnosis – once you know you are suffering from panic attacks you know the worst that can happen to you. So regardless of how severe the symptoms are, you can remind yourself that panic attacks are non-life threatening - that you can revive. Hang on tight and focus on emptying your mind – try and think of NOTHING.

Why diagnosis is good for you

Furthermore, diagnosis does not mean the end of the road. Diagnosis often amounts to a cross-road; you will need to decide what the next step is, for you to continue your journey in life. Strangely enough, once you are faced with no choice but to face the diagnosis, many options that you have never thought would be possible tend to reveal themselves to you.

When I was at the early stage of facing huge daily panic attacks, I was always wondering about how I could move on. Prior to my panic condition, I had always thought I would stay in one job in one company just like family members of my father's generation did until retirement. I thought golden rice bowls existed. But the fact is, times have changed. There are no golden rice bowls. In fact, as fast as a phone changes in trend with better technology, so do our jobs. We are easily dispensable. When one nerve in your body snaps to cause you immobility, you become history.

Despite the high level of stress, I was actually comfortable with my career. Yet, the minute I succumbed to my illness, my job prospects were over.

It is important, actually, to accept this as a fact of life – there is no security of employment, so it is useful to make plans even when there is no diagnosis hanging over you. Developing a habit of positive mentality *to expect the unexpected* with regards to life and having backup plans laid out *prior to needing a plan* could make a difference in moving forward. An unprepared mind will cloud all positive possibilities that can happen to you.

If you choose to be negative about a diagnosis, you will never discover the golden opportunities and rewards that are on the way for you. The rewards come with every struggle of the painful journey we go through. For example, previously, prior to diagnosis, your life might have been so busy that you were never able to enjoy quality time with your loved ones. However, with diagnosis, the process of recovery itself could bring about closer ties and stronger bonds with your loved ones. You can never buy quality time. It is priceless.

Happiness

Sometimes, our mind is so occupied with the stresses of earning money to survive that we tend to relate happiness to the amount of money we earn. Actually, happiness can come without the need of much money. People living in slums can still be happy. Happiness comes from the heart and the ability to love. With lots of money and without the heart to love and, more importantly, the time to love, life gradually becomes very lonely. This is not to say that rich people cannot be happy, but I have noticed that the ones who are happy are so not because they have a lot money but due to the inner peace that they have developed by focusing on achieving a quality life. Such people will not lose their peace even if they lose their material wealth.

The speed and level of recovery depends entirely on the individual. It is up to you to decide to live in denial of the diagnosis or seek help to recover. I must confess that, within my inner self, I was initially very much in denial before I had full blown panic attacks. Deep inside I knew the stresses that I went through at work were killing my soul. Yet I ignored the symptoms even when they caused me extreme discomfort. I thought that everybody suffered some kind of stress and that it was unnecessary for me to talk about my concerns. I was afraid that I would sound like a whiner.

My diagnosis, however, has changed my thinking about life. When situations change, so do dreams. When I thought I was in control of my life prior to my diagnosis, I overlooked many things that could have led me to a happier life. Hence, I could not see and understand the meaning and beauty behind the diagnosis immediately when suddenly my life slipped beyond my control.

One great barrier to acceptance and recovery is the EGO - you need to Eliminate E to GO forward. In other words, accept your diagnosis and move on. After all, recovery begins with YOU. You are the ultimate decision maker with regards to accepting the diagnosis. In fact, this acceptance has to happen before any professional or caregiver can even begin to offer their help to you.

The road to recovery - teamwork

Recovery is actually a teamwork affair. It is not an individual journey but one with a team of supporting travellers. This is the time you learn how to express yourself, discover the potentials in you, accept who you are, eliminate the burdensome baggage of the past, plan for the future and learn how to achieve small goals that lead the way to bigger goals that can be achieved.

Successful people accept facts and are willing to do what unsuccessful people refuse to do. The recovery journey brings you to a new life and a new reality check. For a building to remain solid, a strong foundation is crucial. It is the same with life. Balancing one's life is key. There is no one who can build that foundation but you. In any situation of life, we have to make many decisions. Small decisions and huge decisions. Regardless of the size of the decision, it starts with you. For an example, in daily life, we need food. We eat because a team of messengers inside your body sends a signal to your brain its need for food. Ultimately, who decides? You. You decide if you want to accept the information from the brain and eat, or whether you will remain hungry. When your brain chooses to respond positively to the information, it will start exploring menus that will satisfy your body, the eyes will look for the necessary ingredients, the hands will do the washing, chopping and cooking, and the mouth will do the eating. Your body gets satisfied. The same goes with diagnosis. Whatever the diagnosis may be, a conscious decision to accept and move on has to be made.

The road to recovery – taking your time

You decide where you want to go and when – at your own pace and time. There must be no datelines for recovery, especially for panic and anxiety disorders. Rush would only worsen your condition and contribute an added stress.

When driving, if you wish to avoid dangers on the road, you do not want to rush too much to reach your destination. Similarly, when eating, you do not want to eat too fast such that you fail to enjoy the taste and texture of the food. The same goes for recovery.

The rush for recovery is something to be entirely avoided. You recover only for yourself, for you to see and feel the difference.

Setting your targets according to other people's expectations can be hazardous.

For me, only after three years of unemployment as a result of being ill was I able to believe in myself again. Before that my tunnel vision hindered me from seeing opportunities. I was too busy looking for the causes that led me to become sick, and wondering why they had to happen to me.

Then at one point, I realised it was pointless to worry about causes that were beyond my control. The words from my final boss had scarred me so much that I had plunged into deep depression. After three years, I saw that the diagnosis was an opportunity to break free from her. It finally occurred to me that the loss was not mine as I had always done my best to ensure every job was done. A ridiculous expectation that had a potential to ruin your mind and body was totally not worth committing to. I realised that greed for money could set off vicious cycles.

When I opened my mind to understand my condition and diagnosis, I saw the light at the end of the tunnel. I believe now that God gave me temporary darkness so that I can see all lights more clearly. Sometimes, when everything is too clear in life, we forget about the blind spots of our life. We forget what we really need in life. My world suddenly came into total darkness with the diagnosis. And, somehow, in that darkness I began understanding what I really wanted in life.

Whether or not you ultimately recognise the food item itself, you will be amazed at how much you learn using your taste buds, sense of smell and brains instead of your sight. You will find that you have to take things slower and put things into perspective because you are using your other senses to appreciate the food, not just sight.

God blesses us with different unique senses for us to utilise and this is what makes life beautiful. Therefore, when you are faced with the darkness of a diagnosis to accept, do activate your other senses to connect with your heart. Who knows what other blessings and hidden opportunities may emerge with time?

Try this experiment:

- Blindfold yourself.
- Get someone to feed you something unusual.
- See if you can figure out what it is. The heart connects more strongly with the mind compared

to a vivid eyesight. Just like performing prayers, Yoga or meditation, where you have to close your eyes to disconnect from your current surroundings and achieve an inner peace deep within you.

Accepting diagnosis

In accepting diagnosis, I have learnt to accept myself as well. After all, pain changes people. You learn to understand your body's and mind's limitations. Even though I had lost my first home – one in which I had invested so much emotional currency, lost my source of income after being ill, and also lost my savings by not working for three years, I realised that GOD has given me quality time for myself instead.

Solitude has helped me many times to cope when circumstances get out of control at my end, thanks to my will power to fight every challenge that arose during my recovery journey. Somehow, from that solitude, I wrote and produced a music album entitled "Solitude". In my personal experiences of solitude, I began to appreciate the quality time just being myself within myself.

I strongly believe GOD listened and understood me well. HE knows I was not appreciated for my efforts. So, I needed a break from the vicious cycle. I did not open my eyes to read the writings on the wall. And so, things had to happen so that I could lead a better life.

I made a decision to write this book because I realised that not many people are aware of the consequences of not being able to cope with stress and the destructive side effect of panic attacks. The immediate consequence of being unable to cope with stress is that you can lose your job. If you do not have savings or invested in properties, or have a new job to move to, such a stress can evolve into a living nightmare.

Thus, always put your welfare as your first priority so that you can move on in life. You are the first pillar of decision-making for survival. With diagnosis, patience must follow. When we lose certain things in life but choose to develop patience and a great attitude, you may be rewarded with a gratifying feeling that you have to experience in order to appreciate. And you can inspire others when you display such an attitude.

Overcoming fears

Panic or anxiety disorder diagnosis itself will create a panic for first timers or caregivers who had never heard or encountered such a term. My doctor told me it is quite a common condition, but, most times, when I share my situation, people seem to be ignorant of the existence of this mental issue. They do not know how to help. That is also one reason I force myself to share these facts from my experiences – I strongly feel that it is imperative that someone creates awareness so that prevention is possible. Prevention is always better than cure.

Panic attack is a manifestation of overwhelming fear. It is important that we register the definition about FEAR to help us manage fear better.

F - False
E - Evidence`
A - Appearing
R - Real

When the situation was so bad for me that I began hallucinating, I had to keep telling myself that what I saw was simply false evidence appearing real and that it would eventually fade away. As a matter of fact, hallucinations are indeed unreal. We know it. Circumstances lead me to experiencing situations. Once when I just could not get adequate sleep, I encountered hallucinations of my bedroom being filled with growing metallic branches. It was a phenomenal encounter. I knew at the back of my mind that it was not real but I was too overwhelmed with depression to counter the hallucination. I felt that were too many things happening at the same time for too many times more than I was able to deal with. I felt choked with the amount of information I had to process in the little time and space I had to breathe. This is what happens when underlying issues are not dealt with and left to sleep for years. It is like an erupting volcano. Magmas of fears and anger built up over time that is hot enough to explode.

Now I know that I need to put my fears into a box and throw away the key for good. Forgetting our fears or ignoring them is not sufficient. It has to be faced and overcome. Overloaded fears result in panic because small fears will eventually lead to huge fears.

Don't blame yourself

Do remember that depression, panic and anxiety attacks are not signs of weakness. Do believe and accept that it is actually a testament that you have had to be strong for too long a time. Do know that it is a temporary phase, to force you to rest your mind, body and soul.

Our life journey is like a jigsaw puzzle. Anyone who has ever fixed a jigsaw puzzle would understand and agree that the process of solving the puzzle entails great perseverance, especially for the challenging parts of the picture. Many years back, when I was steady and well, I remember setting a goal to put together thousands of small pieces of jigsaw puzzle to complete the picture of Winnie the Pooh as a gift to my best friend, Azlina, for her first born. My goal was to complete and present her when she gave birth. I had never tried fixing a jigsaw all my life and was not sure about the process of accomplishing it. I was not prepared for any obstacles. All I knew was that I had visualised that I could because it would make my best friend happy. I was not thinking so much of the process but I was focussed on the results. And I did make it on time. But I managed because I had help. She went into the labour ward when I was only halfway done. Nevertheless, my siblings and even my parents helped, and my goal was achieved.

Similarly, after my diagnosis broke my own life into many tiny pieces, I chose to see it as a jigsaw puzzle and chose to get my family to help in piecing it together. I know the process may not always be easy and smooth sailing, but I know I can make things work out.

Welcome the struggle

This reminds me of the story of a boy and a cocoon, a classic example of why struggles can be good.

The Boy and the Butterfly

Once, a little boy was playing outdoors and he found a caterpillar. He was fascinated with the beauty of nature and sought permission from his mother to keep the caterpillar. His mum allowed him, provided the boy promised to take good care of it.

The little boy was happy, put the little 'worm' into a jar and fed it with fresh leaves regularly. Time passed and, one day, the caterpillar climbed up a stick in the jar and started to create a cocoon. His mother explained to the little boy about metamorphosis and how the caterpillar would soon transform into a butterfly. Excited, the boy observed the process and was eager to see the butterfly emerging from the cocoon.

The day emerged when he noticed that there was a small hole in the cocoon and that the butterfly was struggling to emerge. To help make the process easier, the boy grabbed a pair of scissors and snipped the cocoon to enlarge the hole to assist the butterfly to emerge easily.

Unfortunately, the butterfly that emerged had a swollen body, and small and sadly shrivelled wings. The butterfly was not able to expand its wings to fly. In fact, the butterfly ended with defects such that it was not able to fly, it could only crawl about.

Out of curiosity, the little boy's mother brought him to talk to an expert on butterflies. They learned that the butterfly was **supposed** to have struggled to come out of the cocoon. By struggling, the butterfly would have pushed fluid out of its body into its wings. The boy had, in rushing to 'help' the butterfly emerge without effort actually hampered its development permanently. That poor butterfly would never be able to fly and would never be as beautiful as it could have been.

As in the above story, I have learnt that struggling is an important part of **any** growth experience. As a human being, we should never stop growing and expanding our mind. There is a difference in thinking between someone who decides to get well and someone who merely frets over the reasons his health has deteriorated until it is too late to get help. By choosing to struggle and solve our problems, we may be able to develop the ability to fly just like a butterfly, and move on to the consequent chapters of our lives.

Another thing to remember: a diagnosis on your mental condition is not much different from a diagnosis on any other serious medical condition. Only through acceptance, the next step of procuring a better and happier life in a long or short period of time can be achieved. My beloved mum never failed to remind me with love and support to accept my diagnosis, from day one when I was unwell. Her advice was priceless: "Treat it as if you have a cold. Have medication and plenty of water to rest. Tomorrow is a new day."

I am fortunate to have such an amazing woman for a mother. She is one of the reasons I am inspired to constantly choose to be better. She is one strong lady with an iron will. She also reminds me to always pray for a clear clean heart, and that when I do something, to do it sincerely with focus.

In addition to all the struggles that she has had thrown to her throughout her life, caring for me has been an additional one. Yet she has remained strong because she accepted my diagnosis with a clear heart before I did.

She has had a lot to carry on her plate but she did it stoically because she believes in accepting what is fated. While some choose suicide, or to sit around and mope about catastrophes, she chooses to believe life can only get better after overcoming the worst. We do not grow when things are easy. We only grow when we face challenges.

Reflections

- Accepting a diagnosis is not easy but is an essential step to recovery.
- That recovery can only be achieved by embracing the help others offer you, but also by believing in yourself and being prepared to struggle.
- If you have a positive attitude, you will not only recover, you may actually be able to progress further and achieve more of your potential than if you continued just surviving in the stressful world you lived in before your body and mind forced you to stop.
- In other words, the diagnosis may actually turn out to be the best thing that happened to you!

FOUR

Decisions and willingness to be helped

Throughout life, we are continuously making decisions. Sometimes, these are done consciously after considering all known factors. Sometimes, the decision itself is subconscious and we ourselves are not aware that we have chosen our path. The fact is we are constantly making decisions that will determine what happens next. We decide what to do the moment we wake up daily. To brush our teeth first or to shower first. To make the bed first or to roll around the mattress a little bit longer especially on weekends, where, for some, there is no need to rush for work. As the day goes by, decisions after decisions start to work its way naturally into our lives until we decide to end our day with rest. Isn't it amazing just how many decisions we have to make even on the most routine day!

As I pointed out in the earlier chapter, one of the most important decisions you have to make once you accept diagnosis is to allow others to help you. No number of doctors or support groups, no amount of medicine can help if a patient with panic disorder cannot make that decision.

Acceptance of diagnosis is the first huge step. The decision to be helped is the next huge one.

Some will choose to keep their diagnosis purely personal and confidential. I can understand the reason why as I felt the same way when I was first diagnosed; I felt lost, confused, worried about the speculations that would arise, and most importantly, about how others were going to look down on me. Believe me, this unhealthy concern is the one that should never be in our thoughts. Period. Despite efforts to create awareness, there is always a stigma attached when a person decides to get help from a mental health institution. The mental hospital where I lived did not just treat severe psychotic cases but also other conditions relating to the mind, including obsessive compulsive disorder, schizophrenia, panic conditions, dementia, etc.

There are many categories of mental illness and needing treatment does not mean we are stark mad and a danger to society. The institution where I seek treatment is constantly renovated to create a very healthy and nice ambience for visits. Subsidised fees patients enjoy luxurious space and services as much as a private patient. It is almost like a mall with various amenities. In other words, it is similar to the local general hospitals. Yet, people baulk at being seen at a mental institution.

The definition of mental institution creates fear in the minds of the public. I was one of them.

Initially, I thought it was shameful to enter a mental institution for treatment as I did not want to be labelled "mentally ill". I knew that my depression was getting out of control and that I had not been able to recognise myself most times. To uphold my reputation, I sought help from a private psychologist, which eventually cost me a bomb due to the fact that I was unemployed and I kept dipping into my savings to pay for session after session with a private psychologist.

The private psychologist also did not keep a central record system to which other professionals could easily refer – this was the other drawback of my initial decision. This is because other professionals whose help I needed did not have access to my records, which was important for continuity in follow-ups.

Nevertheless, throughout the private psychologist consultations, I made efforts to recover. I listened intently to what could be done to help myself because time was precious and so was money; the consultations were definitely not cheap. My goal was to rush my recovery so that I could move on with life as soon as possible. I treated mental illness like my livelihood in the corporate world: rush and get it done.

Role of a psychologist

Of course, there are no shortcuts to any kind of success, and that includes recovery. Nevertheless, there was progress in that I learnt how to express myself and discuss underlying issues with the psychologist.

I was new to the idea of speaking to a psychologist and I was frequently irritated when the psychologist kept asking questions followed by constant nodding and even more questions and nods. I thought I paid money so that I could get answers, but all I received were questions. I failed to understand the unique process of such a treatment. I felt that they were doubtful of me with consistent questions thrown at me.

It was only after I shared my frustrations with one of my sisters (she studied psychology) that I understood that psychologists are actually trained to do this, to help clients open up to the underlying issues we faced.

And then, I came across and read a book entitled "Questions are the Answers" by Allan Pease and it made sense to me. If the psychologist offered solutions and options, I might have objected to them. Questioning me persistently, on the other hand, would eventually lead me to my own options and solutions. No one likes to be told what to do. Therefore, questions were the best mode for answers.

Once I understood the style of treatment, I became more cooperative in answering questions, which gradually probed deeply into my underlying issues. It seemed like a long tiring journey southward to find the lost Titanic ship buried underwater for the longest time. I was astonished to find that I had so much to talk about and discuss. One step at a time, discoveries were made and layer after layer of my memories were peeled and examined.

I realised that I could work out my own solutions, but I need the help of a professional to ask the right questions.

I had to learn how to trust a professional who, despite being a stranger, was able and willing to help. I needed to be willing to have an open honest discussion no matter how dark my past was.

The advantage of trained professionals over friends and family is their objectivity - there is no emotional reaction in their desire to help me.

Do something!

However, again, after we come up with solutions, implementing them depends entirely on us. We can choose to sit for another 100 years on the **Actions** that need to be addressed after discussion with the psychologist, but then we would be wasting time. When that mentality persists, nothing new will happen. We will end up doing the same thing and expecting a different result. Nothing ventured, nothing gained.

Have you ever listened to someone who constantly shared with you the same problem time after time, year after year? But, when you suggest a solution, nothing gets done to make things better or at least provide some room for improvement?

I know of someone who has been griping about his situation for many years now. I have since overcome so many different and difficult obstacles in life but his problem still remains unsolved. The fact is he has been indulging in self-pity rather than trying to find a solution. A vicious cycle then develops, the more he whines the harder it becomes to get out of the rut. He needs to decide to take action, only then can things change.

Recovery involves a huge amount of **COURAGE** and **WILLPOWER**. If you cannot commit to getting better, you will never get better. You have all the power to change things. In fact, I believe that the people who have experienced the worst past and yet choose to move forward are the ones who end up creating the best futures. In business, the successful ones are the ones who dare to take huge bold risks for a bigger success. In the highly competitive entertainment show business, those who survive over years and still have the 'pull' factor are those who constantly reinvent themselves – these are the ones who are willing to learn and constantly grow in thinking.

In short, the difference between hugely successful people and unsuccessful ones is mainly in the way they **THINK**. It all starts with super strong dreams. So strong that no one can take that dream away. This dream in not simply a sleeping dream that passes with wakefulness but a solid rock dream that can withstand the many rejections and objections that will surely crop up along the way to success.

Intelligence does not in itself assure anything if it is not used to make plans that emerge from the strong dream, and then effort is committed into implementing these plans. I am not born with the kind of amazing intelligence that allows some to top their classes without studying. I had to study hard to achieve simple achievements when schooling.

People who do not have to study and yet excel in school seem lucky – they are subject to little pressures. But this is not necessarily a good thing. I have always admired a friend of mine who was so intelligent that he excelled in school. Yet, one day, he told me that he was not ambitious and had no burning desire to do something out of the ordinary. I was amazed. In my heart, intelligence without drive to reach the skies is a shameful waste. With intelligence as his gift from GOD, he could have reached financial freedom at a young age, he could have been an influential leader, he could have been a motivational speaker, he could have done so much to contribute to society: but he did nothing make his mark once he left school. Was that not a pity?

On the other hand, without being born with a super intelligent brain, my perspective in life had always been different. I was willing to struggle to achieve small goals. And I had dreams. I envision a life where financial freedom is achieved at a reasonably young age so that one has the option to retire and secure the freedom of time to do what is worth doing. When you achieve both goals you are able to help others. If not you get stuck trading every single second of your life for a few dollars.

I remember vividly the day an ex-flatmate of mine – a manager who conducted interviews to employ personnel for the food and beverage department – returned home feeling dejected. He shared to me that he was deeply saddened that one of his applicants was a 70-year-old man applying for the position of kitchen helper. Is 70 years still not enough to stop trading time for money? I was saddened by the fact too.

Upon hearing to the plight of the 70-year-old man, I began to ponder the possibilities and consequences of the decisions I would eventually have to make with regards to my mental health. I was undergoing depression at the time. Even so, the facts below screamed out to me:

- I could choose to work towards wellness or remain in denial about my mental health situation.
- I could choose to seek early treatment or simply sit on my underlying issues.
- I could work towards some goal or just wallow in self-pity.

In other words, I could choose to move one step forward or remain where I was forever. Thank goodness God had not taken away my thinking cap and ability to decide. By questioning and answering my inner self on the next step, naturally, my conscious mind went into the next choice of what I could choose to do in order to enjoy a different, better life.

I pressed on and asked myself what would happen if I were to lose my mind completely but my body was still alive – the prospect of having to trouble my loved ones with the expense of my upkeep was horrifying. I realised it would be selfish of me to give in to my circumstances instead of taking the chance of choosing to survive.

Prior to making a decision to survive, the first thing that came across my mind was my ageing parents. My dad is in his 60s and my mum, her 50s. They are both survivors. My three siblings and I had witnessed with our very own eyes how many times they fell and then picked themselves up.

At 34, I was certainly facing some serious predicaments, but so did they when they were at my age. Panic disorder meant that my body and my mind were at odds with one another with deep depression and severe anxieties. By right, both mind and body should be balanced. Unfortunately, mine were having a crisis with each other and were in a war zone. Making decisions was even harder than before. Just like our personal computers, at times, when overused, it needs to be rebooted a few times to work well again. Similarly, with my brain. As my brain gets rebooted each time I see a psychologist, I recognised that a psychologist was indeed crucial in my move forward. This is because every time I decide to trust my issues with people who had an emotional attachment with me, the most common response was the reassurance that my problems and issues were not too serious; that many other people faced much bigger issues. Statements like that are very destructive - just how big must an issue be before people will accept I am likely to lose my mind? How long should I totally ignore issues? Because of such statements, I totally ignored my underlying issues for too long a time; I believed wrongly that my problems were never too serious for me to seek help.

I was glad that God triggered the faces of my parents in my mind when I had to make a decision. I would always want to provide the best for my parents as they have provided their best for me. They believed in my recovery before I did. Support from loved ones is indeed helpful. Nevertheless, even if you think that you do not have the support of close relatives or friends for your recovery, you still have to make the choice to be a survivor. Choose to be well for yourself because it is you who gain most from such a decision.

Be aware, however, that the decision to recover and to accept help will not magically change your life. The road to recovery is an arduous one, possibly fraught with many more challenges to overcome before you can claim the mystery prize.

In the following pages, I will try to outline some of the immediate challenges that came my way.

Fear of the outside

Agoraphobia was a huge challenge. With unemployment and as a side-effect of antidepressants, my fear of the outside world heightened. I craved silence and to be by myself. The only outdoors for me was standing by the window and admiring for a short moment the beauty of trees and watching the sunrise and sunset. I became one of my domestic pussycats. A big pussycat indeed with a long tail of underlying issues to figure out and settle.

And so, during the days of my deep depression where I stood by the window gazing into the thin air, I was totally unable to muster the courage to exit the premises of my home. My home was comfortable and it provided me a safe sanctuary, but getting out of the house was still of vital importance.

The solution

One morning, while being severely depressed and standing by the window, something caught my attention, and triggered some hope in me. A neighbour was walking with his dog. Shortly after, I saw another resident jogging with his dog. As an animal lover who cares for all species and breeds alike, I was mesmerised and began smiling in spite of myself. That realisation made me ponder - how about walking a dog to fight my fear of going out of the house?

More problems

Just the prospect of it made my head spin for many days. I started to tremble and shake ridiculously out of the fear that cynophobes (people who fear dogs) would be afraid of approaching me. Also, Muslims traditionally do not keep dogs and I was afraid members of my community might condemn me without understanding my need.

I was even more fearful of the dog-walking idea because I was fully aware how vulnerable I was as a consequence of the ease with which I connected with animals. I feared that creating a bond with a dog might lead to more problems, as I was unemployed and already had six cats to feed. I got by only because God had sent me a wonderful housemate, Charles, who had by then not only understood how serious my problems were, but had also proceeded to become my immediate caregiver. It was he who now paid the rent fully and even paid for my cats' food. I could not see how I could burden him further.

These overwhelming fears triggered severe panic attacks day after day because I was not able to communicate my thoughts and concerns.

How I wished I could walk my well-fed home-loving pussies! It would have been such an easy solution then. Unfortunately, the dear critters did not share my need for the outdoors!

I felt I was as good as a blind man who needed a guide dog to move around, and in my case, just to breathe the air outside again.

Isn't it ironical? I was already beset with so much panic before I even possessed a dog. A simple sight from my window created so much distress to my body and mind. Just like that, I snapped and went bonkers.

That was how dire my situation was. Even as I sought solutions to every problem that came my way, I would freak out thinking about the pros and cons of each solution. I felt like running away from my solutions. I was totally out of control despite making a conscious decision to be a survivor and recover.

Mustering courage

I suppose those journeys were part of the process that I had to undergo and had to keep on fighting till I won the battle. Not many who knew me knew what I went through in fighting the depression battle. I was fighting all alone during the day.

I began praying emotionally to God requesting further guidance from Him as to my next step. Night prayers are special to me as it is the time where everything goes silent. It is the time when the connection between God and me seems strongest. I always seek His light to show me a way out of my dilemmas.

Thereafter, I somehow managed to share with Charles the reasons for the deterioration of my condition. We had a long discussion about the whole idea. He stated that he was already looking for ways to break my agoraphobia. His goal was for me to take small steps to at least get out of the house and walk around the guarded condominium territory if not totally out into the real world. If I did not take these steps, I would never be able to go back to the real world.

Charles used to have dogs, one of which had passed on while the other had been given out for adoption due to personal reasons. He reminded me that a dog came with huge responsibilities. He was also fearful of my unstable and vulnerable condition.

To strengthen my willpower for positive thinking, I recited in my heart prayers and affirmed my intention that I intended to walk a dog purely to minimise my overwhelming agoraphobia and improve my focus on walking out again, in the name of GOD. I kept reciting and re- affirming it over and over to calm my anxieties.

In the midst of all these tribulations, Charles surprised me one day and brought home a tiny three-month-old shih- tzu puppy. He looked like the "Ewok" character from Star Wars. Charles named him "Monty".

Charles made me promise not to worry so much about other people's opinion of Monty as, officially, Monty belonged to him and not me, if my fear was the condemnation of people who did not understand.

Charles reckoned that I could help him to be a caregiver to Monty by walking him daily. He chose a puppy because he knew I needed time to accept, bond with and understand Monty before the two of us would be ready to face the outdoor world. He hoped that Monty would heal my wounds and get me well again. It was not immediately that I got a chance to walk Monty as he was also too young and afraid. While fostering Monty and waiting for him to grow bigger and stronger, a part of me began healing as I occupied my time well. Days where I was drowned by fears were replaced with some activity involving keeping Monty clean and healthy.

Charles knew that each time I had a new cat, I would be happier and give the best quality care I could. But this time, it was a different and unique new arrival.

Not many knew about me fostering Monty. I only shared with certain people whom I trusted not to look down on me. I had already received several negative comments about my cats, from people who judged based on their numbers and not the way I cared for my kitty kids.

Back to square one

One day, my fear of discrimination was actually realised. A Caucasian condominium resident at our rented apartment stopped Monty and me from walking with his motorbike. He warned me that he never wanted to see me walking Monty ever again as he hated dogs. Shocked, I had a severe panic attack and was sent to the mental hospital for treatment.

And so, all the months of therapies went to waste as I was in depression mode again. This time, however, due to the fact that Monty was so adorable, he healed the wound very quickly. In fact, he still gets me up every time I fall.

There was another episode where a person in whom I entrusted the secret of fostering Monty suddenly decided not to understand the situation and advised me to get well as soon as possible so that I could part with Monty. I had a choking panic attack the moment I read the text message in the middle of a busy road. This time however, even though I was disappointed, I managed to get over the attack without visiting the hospital.

The mysterious process of recovery is not easily understood. Charles gave me a responsibility that suited my condition and gave me the hope of controlling the entire gamut of negative feelings I had: suicidal thoughts, loneliness, depression, anxieties, etc. My small task was just to take good care of Monty, not to think about speedy recovery. People expected me to set a timeline for me to achieve this, when such pressure actually worsens my condition.

Monty

Below is Monty at three months, the first day he arrived and began me on my journey to recovery.

Monty at 3 months old

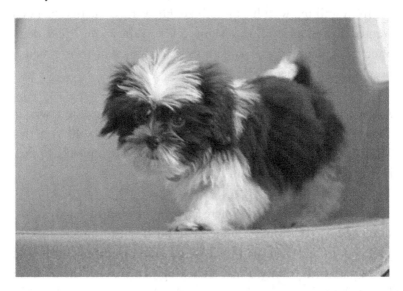

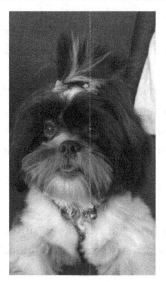 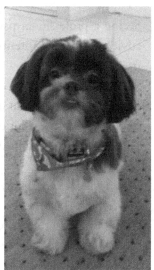

Monty's hairstyle 1   Monty's Hairstyle 2

My cats and Monty are now best of friends. Monty has no idea that he is a pooch. He thinks that he is a cat and still does. He possesses a unique character of constantly wanting to protect me. He knows when I am depressed and he knows when I have a panic attack. He sits next to me each time I have panic attacks and provide me with a positive aura as a lifeline to hang on. He follows me everywhere I go in the house and, somehow, when I have a purpose to my life, my suicidal thoughts naturally subside. I am now able to focus on my prayers more and when I pray, Monty respects my space and time with God. What a pity that some people still do not understand that my full-time therapist in my fight against agoraphobia is a canine!

Reflection

- The decision to take steps towards recovery is only the beginning. Expect to face many more challenges on the way.

- Seeing a professional psychologist is better than receiving advice from well-intentioned but emotionally subjective friends or family.
- When you decide upon a solution for a particular problem, do not let the judgment of ignorant people hinder you from implementing the solution.
- God is Merciful and hears your prayers. Seek His guidance when you feel lost.
- When you face a setback, do not despair – just pick up where you left off.
- Consider getting a pet to help you heal if you suffer from anxiety attacks or depression. They offer unconditional love and are always available.

FIVE

The Power of Breathing and Mindfulness

Everybody knows that without oxygen, we cannot breathe. However, sometimes, we are so occupied with our troubles that we forget to breathe even when the air is clean and fresh. We only realise the importance of breathing when we can no longer breathe normally. In 2013, Singapore and Malaysia came under the blanket of one of the worst haze in decades. Due to forest fires from a neighbouring country, for a few weeks, the Pollutant Standards Index reached an alarming level of danger, so much so that it was dangerous for us to breathe outdoors. Suddenly, fresh air to breathe became a precious commodity. There was a mad rush to pharmacies looking for protective masks. The acrid reek of smoke was so pervasive it stuck on your clothes. The haze eventually went away but it served a wake-up call for me and many others who experienced the terrifying air quality. It showed just how vital a clean and healthy environment was. Only then did many people become mindful of the serious consequences of environmental pollutants.

Just like the haze stoked mass panic to a small extent, the unhealthy environment of one's mind can cause overwhelming fear to stir up a panic attack in those who are vulnerable, often resulting in hyperventilation. The process of hyperventilation can set off its own vicious cycle, especially for first timers who have never experienced or expected the sudden shortness of breath. There are times where there are no warning signs that the shortness of breath is about to occur. You panic, thinking you will die of breathlessness, which makes you hyperventilate even more!

This is why practicing mindfulness and good breathing techniques is a must for anyone who faces anxiety issues. The technique is simple and it can save your life.

The technique

1. Begin by inhaling and exhaling deeply and fully.
2. As you do so, visualise a blank white canvas.
3. Insert into the blank canvas in your mind any beautiful memories that you have. For example, if you are a parent, this might be something funny your child did. If you are single, one of your former achievements could make a great memory. For animal lovers, there are always the moments when your pet made you laugh - just choose one.
4. With your eyes shut, focus on beautiful memories on the canvas of your mind to temporarily distract the body so that the body can work its way to normality.

Finding a lifeline

I am an animal lover. I include at the end of the chapter some pictures of my babies that keep me breathing. Because of them, I have a purpose in life and a reason to overcome depression. They are my lifeline and hope towards recovery. Finding yourself a lifeline of hope is literally life-saving. Depression can lead to suicidal thoughts and suicidal thoughts can kill you. They should be banished from your mind.

Sometimes, when the going gets tough, it is important that you quickly reflect and identify the lifelines that can encourage you to remain positive. Seek assistance from someone whom you trust so that you can breathe, take one step at a time and return to being mindful of positivity.

There are **NO** problems in life that cannot be solved if you put your mind and heart to find the solution or at least the next step to begin with. Even if you cannot see the possibilities, there are other people who can help you see what you cannot, provided you allow them to help you.

Hold my hand

If you are a caregiver and your loved one is hyperventilating because of his anxieties, you can help. Hold his hands, close your eyes and breathe together. It will not only help the person feeling troubled calm down, but it will also help you feel better.

Breathing out with love

Practising proper breathing daily can improve your quality of life even when you are not unwell. The way you breathe reflects the way you live. Have you ever walked by the beach with the gentle sea breeze caressing your face? As you inhale and exhale deeply, did you not find your stresses fall off like the water off a duck's back? It is a feeling that you wish will not come to end.

Such an experience not only creates contentment but it also acts as a key to the inner peace of your body and mind. The full and free breathing will lift up your spirit and well-being naturally.

It is through breathing that a new-born baby learns to get in touch with the basic rhythm of life. Each breath that we inhale represents the acceptance of the universe and exhaling represents giving back to the universe. When breathing itself is at ease with the right frame of mind, there is no reason to think about the past and worry about the future. Quality breathing clarifies the mind. Whatever your situation may be, no matter how complicated it may seem, even if you have to breathe in with anger, let it out with love. With time and consistent practice, breathing in and out with love without much effort becomes possible.

Each time I breathe to clear my anxieties, I focus on my cats who constantly make me laugh. It has always been a sweet experience. They are my lifeline and I utilise that love to help me with my breathing during my difficult times enduring anxieties and panic conditions.

My cats

I have been blessed with 11 cats, eight boys and three girls. Eight out of the 11 are rescued cats. Honestly, my recovery process would not have been the same without my kitties. They have witnessed my ups and downs and when times were really bad for me, having panic attacks alone at home, they would come to me and offer their bodies for me to hug so that we could breathe together.

When I have a breathing crisis, closing my eyes and hugging one of my kitties and following its breathing pace helps me breathe properly.

Mario and Luigi were my first adopted kitties from the pet rescue shelter. Seven years ago, I made a commitment to love them and that love has never run out. Prior to succumbing to the anxiety disorder, Mario and Luigi were the support I needed when I thought I could not do it. They have licked my tears, slept with me and checked on me in bed to make sure I was breathing, so that I could feed them.

When it comes to mealtimes in the morning, the first thing they would do is check if I am alive by rubbing and putting their faces close to mine.

Luigi has turned out to be a fat cat. These two siblings have their routines where Mario would check on me in the morning and once Mario acknowledges to Luigi that I am still alive, fat cat Luigi will sit on my chest to wake me up for food. Luigi puts on his "Puss in boots" face. How could I ever resist such charms? Never.

When I feel horrible as a result of medical drug side effects and anxieties, hugging fat cat Luigi definitely helps ease the pain tremendously. I bet he knows that his human daddy needs him.

Mindfulness

With panic attacks, we do experience tunnel vision. In other words, we tend to focus exclusively on our emotions. As a result, perception becomes selective and we have difficulty seeing things clearly. Such a situation will lead us to being blind toward our hopes and dreams. With their unconditional love, my pussycats nudge my mind to positivity again and remind me to be mindful of the good things around me.

Attaining mindfulness simply means developing a state of mind that is stable and calm. Since panic is the antithesis of calm, mindfulness is certainly not easy to achieve during a panic attack, but it is not impossible. With practice, we can achieve anything.

It took me a while to master the art and skill of mindfulness even though my pussycats were there physically. I was too occupied with the pain and discomfort of anxieties. I knew that my pussycats loved and needed me but I was also unable to control my emotions because of the fears I had in me. My pussycats were in a better state of mindfulness compared to me.

The moment I achieved the skill of being mindful, certain things that I had been previously blind to slowly emerged and became more apparent.

I had been afraid to get out of my apartment. The sound of vehicles on the road and people irritated me. I was afraid to hear the opinions of other people. Suicidal thoughts were natural.

Now that my mindfulness is stronger than negativity, I am myself amazed that I was tempted by suicide. No matter how low I feel, I acknowledge my compassion for the cats forces me to rethink my options.

Mario and Luigi always know when I need them badly. I need not call them - both boys will approach me. Mario will sit on my lap while Luigi spreads his legs to distract me. He will be like, "Hey! Look here! Stop being depressed. You've got a tummy to rub! Come on, I'm waiting!" And if I don't pay attention, Luigi will wriggle his body and sway his head left to right seeking attention. He is persistent and never gives up on me. Sometimes, the rest will join in. Alejandro, the black cat, is a kissing cat. It will kiss my lips to break me out of my daze of deep thoughts.

The thing about cats is that you do not own them but they own you. They are the bosses of my household. I see it as my duty to provide them with great quality food and a clean home environment and they give me a sense of purpose to still be alive. Cats are intelligent creations of God. They are fully aware of situations and taking care of me was equally important to them.

Cats themselves are very good when it comes to mindfulness of surroundings and situations. There is so much to learn from Mother Nature.

Cats eat, sleep, play and stretch. Stretching was something I did not do. Eating and sleeping were things I could not enjoy when I was depressed. What more to play or relax my mind with activities that I loved to do! Cats taught me the basics of a calm lifestyle.

While waiting for me to complete my morning prayers, my cats would usually hang around my prayer mat and chill out. They know that after prayer is breakfast for them. Seated on my prayer mat and observing them play, suddenly, my mind was clear and for a moment I could figure out what I needed to do. I began to see a little light at the end of the tunnel. Previously, I was always caught up with the urgency of recovering speedily so that I could start earning an income of my own. My savings were drying up and everyone around me always wished me a speedy recovery. I felt I had a deadline to meet.

I suppose speedy recoveries are a good thing for physical illness conditions. For mental illnesses, however, hoping for a quick recovery can have adverse effects. We cannot rush recoveries. It is not a sprint race but a lifetime marathon. In rushing recovery, relapse becomes a greater possibility.

That was the mistake I consistently made, the rush to recover. That fateful morning, my cats made me realise that I needed to work towards eating well, sleeping well, breathing well and stretching my body physically. These are simple healthy actions yet often forgotten or ignored. Just like my happy cats, those exercises somehow worked on my journey towards being my usual self again. My passion for rescuing and fostering animals continues.

Images representing LOVE that reinforce the importance of Mindfulness and Breathing again.

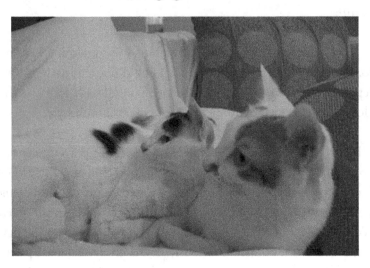

Triki (the one with the black spots)

Triki was a stray kitten. I found her in a car park and saved her from being run over by cars. She was shaken, hungry and very dirty. She is now the DIVA among the boys. The moment she entered my home, it was clear that she was confident that my home was going to be her permanent home. She has no intention of going out anymore.

If cats can choose to be happy and love, so can human beings!

Mario. The leader of the pack. Pussycat Mario is the leader of the clowder and he makes sure that all the other cats, including me, are fine.

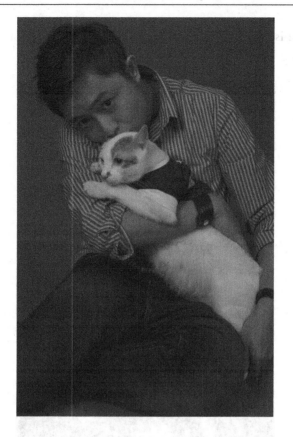

In loving memory of my eldest boy, Luigi, 12 October 2006 to 15 June 2014

He had a huge appetite and he loved to watch me cook. When I washed the dishes, though, he was not interested as food was not involved. Sadly, on 15 June 2014, my eldest boy Luigi passed on. He had a fall, which hit the wrong spot that caused him to be paralysed waist down, and he died unexpectedly 1 day after his paralysis. Luigi was a rescued cat and he lived very well and had been my confidant for my good days and many bad days. He will be deeply missed. Luigi would hug me whenever I had panic attacks so that I could synchronise my hyperventilating mode to the rhythm of his calm breathing.

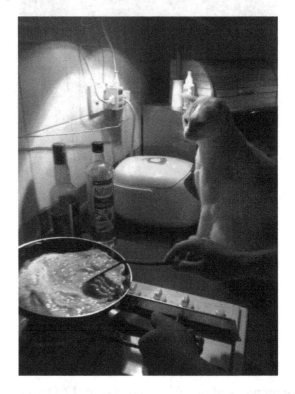

15 June 2014 – The day I lost and bury my eldest furry kid. I quickly swallowed my anti-depressants the moment I heard the sad news on the phone from the animal clinic to calm myself so as to fulfil my final duty as a daddy to Luigi on Father's Day.

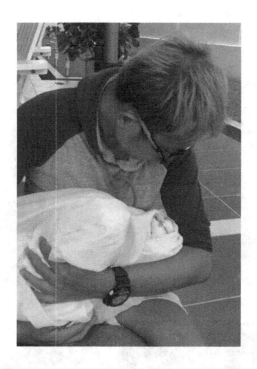

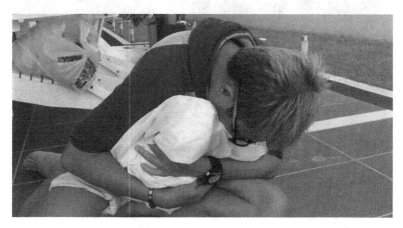

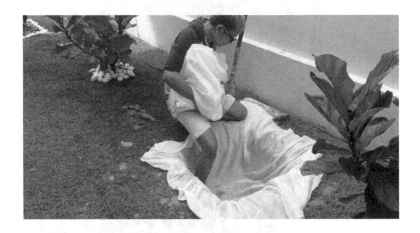

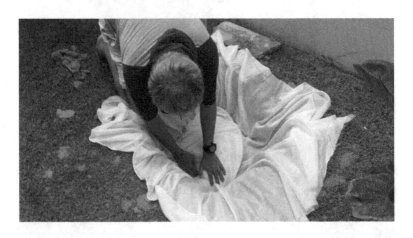

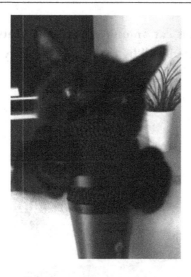

Alejandro, my black kissing cat

Alejandro is the coolest cat among all. He has no tantrums, loves to do a quick kiss on my lips unexpectedly, and is a quiet and independent boy. I have never seen Alejandro in a bad mood. He is the only one that can get along with my most temperamental cat, Triki.

Bubi is my 3-legged cat. He is a special and affectionate cat indeed. He prefers to be left alone most times but comes to me when he needs affection.

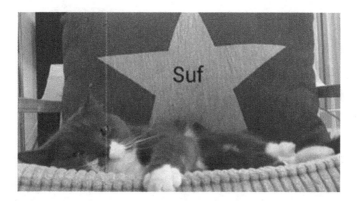

Robby the shyest cat among all my pussycats. Precious and sensitive. Protected well by the rest of the kitty residents.

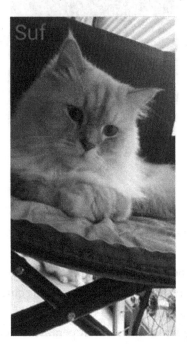

The other five rescued cats (Lucas, Louisa and Chermain, Felix and Charlie Boy) will be featured in Chapter 7.

SIX

Breaking the Vicious Cycle

The cycle of opportunities

The first lesson I remember of my science lessons in primary school is that of the life cycle of a butterfly. I discovered at nine that a caterpillar would eventually transform onto a butterfly. Two totally separate and different lives indeed! Yet, both are beautiful by nature and have their own unique features and qualities. Both need to go through a stage of life that has its own challenges. The crawling land-bound caterpillar has the potential one day to literally fly, and till today I am still amazed by that fact. Life cycles contain opportunities – opportunities for us to grow and move forward into the next step of the cycle. As unique as it is being a butterfly, so are humans who are blessed with a brain to think in order to achieve anything they want to achieve with proper planning and execution of the plan, whatever it may be.

As a toddler, we do not know and cannot imagine that one day we will actually be able to walk, but it comes to most of us with time – we are offered the opportunity to learn step by step to eventually balance, stand and start walking. By nature, anything that has a pulse or life has a cycle to undergo. Frequently, an opportunity in life that comes with a greater potential for fulfilment is also accompanied by more trials and tribulations than we could imagine or think of. There are no shortcuts towards success. We constantly need to strive to fulfil every single goal in life. There are times when the cycle of our opportunities goes smoothly without any glitches and we are happy. Smooth flow of actions leads to satisfaction and personal gain. Just like the sea, when the sea is in a state of calm, the ship sails smoothly. Nevertheless, when the storm arrives, the ship requires extra effort to be stabilised.

Importance of taking steps

Human beings go through storms in the form of rejections, distractions and obstacles to achieve a goal. How we choose to deal with the challenges depends entirely on the way we think. For an example, the difference between a successful entrepreneur and someone who dreams to be one but does not achieve that goal is simply the difference in their "thinking". The way we think has a lot to do with who and what we are going to be. The state of mind determines the way we feel for the day. However, thinking without any actions leads nowhere. Nothing ventured, nothing gained. We can choose to think from now until Christmas but if no actions are taken, we remain where we are. And if actions are still not taken, time continues to move until the next Christmas. So we must take action. Nevertheless, it is always prudent to still think about the pros and cons before we take any important step in any direction.

Recognising vicious cycles

On Fridays, many people tend to feel more relaxed and relieved. Weekends are sought after as they offer the opportunity to spend quality time with either loved ones or to be alone doing things that make you happy. On the other hand, Monday comes with blues because the work week begins. Even when schooling during my teenage years, I used to be depressed on Sundays because I had to go to school the next day. I dreaded sports lessons because I faced discrimination being weaker than the other boys. When I was enlisted to the army for national service, another cycle of fears existed. I feared booking into army camps but I had no choice as it was my compulsory obligation to serve the country. I had several mild to moderate panic attacks during those days but I never recognised them as I had no knowledge of this condition at the time. Once, I had difficulty breathing at the army camp and had cramps all over my face and body. I thought it was merely an asthma attack. With a history of childhood asthma, I knew that wheezing was part of asthma attacks and I had no wheezing during the attack in the army. It was a totally different feeling of breathlessness but I did not understand the significance.

The cycle moved on to working life. Just like everyone else, I felt happiest on Fridays and least happy on Mondays. This became less normal when the stress was so overwhelming that, on Sunday evenings, I would feel all messed up; I feared dealing with stacks of files after files screaming for attention with deadlines to fulfil and facing a boss who only signed documents and expected more to be done, especially bills to clientele. The more you issued bills, the more you were loved. The necessity to remain vigilant with regards to clients' payment of our bills before proceeding to do more urgent work in an environment where rush was part of the game, was very stressful. There were many times on weekends when I returned to work secretly.

What disappointed me most was the lack of recognition; favoured staff were allowed to push their responsibilities to others and yet get the credit and the promotions. As my condition deteriorated, I began thinking more frequently of ways to perfect the way I worked so as to be appreciated. By nature, I was already a perfectionist. The lack of appreciation and being pushed around made me even more obsessed about perfection just to please others. Nevertheless, it was an exercise in futility.

Every time I confess to being a perfectionist, I get the advice, "Chill out, nobody is perfect in this world" or "Perfect is boring". Yet how could I not feel the need to be perfect when I was being constantly compared to others and belittled? My principle in life had always been to improve on constructive criticism to move forward. Unfortunately, the criticism I faced was destructive and I eventually fell deeper into depression, especially with the attitude of my final boss.

In the abyss of depression, I had no control over my worries of not having a roof over my head and having to separate from my beloved pets due to unemployment. I stopped visualising options that could nudge me forward. I felt like screaming at the boss who belittled me. I knew that would be fighting in a ring where I could not win. So I held back because my biggest fear was that of unemployment. On hindsight, I wish I had just been brutally honest about her unacceptable behaviour at the time and lost my job. That would have allowed me to get her out of my mind.

Instead, even today, I still dream of her expressionless and cold face towards me. To cap it all, I ultimately lost my job anyway.

That last boss was inhuman. Knowing that I was vulnerable because I had taken two months' unpaid leave and was on antidepressants, she installed CCTV upon my return to monitor staff movements. I told myself not to panic and to ignore that unfair action.

But she continued making life miserable for me. On returning, I had accepted a downgraded position to reduce my stress. Yet, she would not even smile at me even when I greeted and opened the office door for her. Instead, I was told not to scratch her new wallpaper when seated in the small new desk given to me. Prior to panic attacks, I never had problems of small spaces office – in fact I used to make them into sanctuaries of peace and holistic ambience. But after the medical drugs, I felt choked and claustrophobic within the small space she provided me. And all she cared about was her new wallpaper!

My heart raced as her arrogance escalated further on the same day. She gave me instructions using jargon to pin me down, for example by using "data port" to mean "internet".

As a result of the side effect of antidepressants, I was confused and before I could even attempt to understand what she meant, she raised her voice to represent her condescending tolerance of my stupidity at not understanding her basic commands. Apparently, all she wanted to know was if my internet was working.

When she left, my mind, heart and body all went haywire. I called my friend who was an IT manager to define the word "data port" as I felt so stupid for not having the right frame of mind to counter her weapon of language. I told myself, "This is it! It is time to leave that company and break the vicious cycle." My heart pounded so fast that I excused myself and took a taxi to the mental institution hospital emergency room. Along the way, my limbs went numb and I was struggling hard to breathe normally. I did not want to go back to work. I was petrified. I was not afraid of my boss but I was fed up with the panic attacks she caused me to have.

The unnecessary CCTV installation broke the trust between the management and staff. We felt safer working and were more productive without our tail being stepped on at all times. Nobody likes to be watched all the time. What time you come in, what time you go home and every single move that you make. Privacy and trust gone with the wind just like that.

In the emergency room, I struggled to control my breathing. It took me several hours before I could catch my breath. I regretted spending $300 to beautify my small workspace to inspire myself. I had been ready to start a new working life again after two months of unpaid leave to rest at home. I had made the effort to think positive and see the bright side of life despite being demoted. Yet, one selfish character that had power and money crushed me like a cockroach.

That was the day my depression got worse and when I began to develop agoraphobia. I was in a daze for long hours. I became afraid of many things. I was no longer half the man I used to be. As a formality to exit the company in a good way and with all respect, my best friend, Charles, and my mum requested to meet the belittling boss to explain my situation and request for immediate release. She refused to meet them. In the end, Charles volunteered to claim all my possessions left at the office and the décor items I spent on. I left the company with no proper goodbyes.

Till now, I hate it when she asks my ex-colleagues about me, pretending to be concerned, as if she cannot understand why I went bonkers when I was a good worker. The belittling boss was the biggest cancer and the toughest stain that my mind needed to eliminate. It has been years and I still dream of her. When in the doldrums of depression, I wake up in the middle of the night having difficulties breathing because I dream of her.

Breaking away from oppressive cycles

I had to quit in order to break the vicious cycle that that belittling boss had set in place. Persevering any further would have led me off the cliff. The process of overcoming depression thereafter was a long and winding road. Nevertheless, it was not impossible. Early treatment helped me pull through.

Even though my best friend Charles has always been there to foster my kitty kids and provide me a shelter, my biggest fear is that of losing my best friend.

Uncontrollable negative thoughts like his possible death constantly linger at the back of my head. My direct family members are afraid of cats and I would have to be unjust to either my cats or my family should I lose my best friend and have to return to my family. Each time such thoughts assail me, I get panic attacks.

In panic disorder situations, sometimes, we feel that we have put in so much effort towards recovery; yet there are times we feel that we end up at the same initial spot again. Many times I have felt that all my efforts have gone totally wasted. However, as I continued seeking psychological treatment, gradually I began to see the full picture – I realise that I have actually moved on. First, however, I had to forego my expectations of speedy recovery and learn to appreciate my many small accomplishments during the slow process of recovery. Instead of starting from scratch every time, I set my mind to move on from wherever I had paused.

So, what do I do to eliminate those unnecessary fears each time I face them? In my case, I choose to overcome those fears by prayers and by choosing to strongly believe that everything will be fine. Breaking the vicious cycle requires WILLPOWER to overcome debilitating fears. It is not an easy journey as a slow recovery means many more challenges financially (you not only have no income, your savings will also dry up as you struggle to make do. Add in the cost of regular treatment and you will get a picture of our struggle).

Nevertheless, as long as we have faith in ourselves, God will lead us through, somehow.

I have realised that there are as many kind and sincere people in this world as there are cruel ones who enjoy making you sick. God will show you people who will support you in this fight as long as you try as well and are willing to seek and receive help.

I was good at my job as long as it lasted. I had inspired my colleagues with my ideas of working smart and decorating work spaces with lamps, plants, frames and fish tanks. I was able to offer a shoulder to cry on for anyone who needed it. I was cool, calm and collected. I did not seem to be as frustrated as my other colleagues. Unfortunately, while offering support to others, I inadvertently allowed myself to be emotionally affected too, and I gradually lost grip on my own self-assurance.

Happy survivor or unhappy survivor – your choice

Everyone has problems at work but people do not voice them as freely as they need to because there is no such thing as a golden rice bowl these days. I am amazed at those who have suffered the same problems at work for years but still hold on to their job. On the other hand, I almost lost my mind because I allowed myself to be affected by problems that were not related to me. Sometimes, I wish I could be like them - frustrated yet surviving in a job full of unhappiness. I ask myself, "Why couldn't I be a survivor in that aspect too?"

But then, I also question myself further as to whether that is really what I want. An unhappy survivor? Perhaps by undergoing the process of losing so much, I will one day become a happy survivor instead. I truly believe that is an end worth fighting for. Nevertheless, I remain amazed at their ability to persevere through a vicious cycle for so many years. I think my own mistake was that I was too engrossed and focused on finding solutions to help others be happier working. I was unaware of a critical fact - that there are things in life that is beyond our control. And that, I should not worry about things I cannot control or change. I failed to understand that to be happy, the individual has to make an independent choice to take actions towards such a goal. There was really nothing I could do for others unless they wanted to change things for themselves. I could only do that for myself.

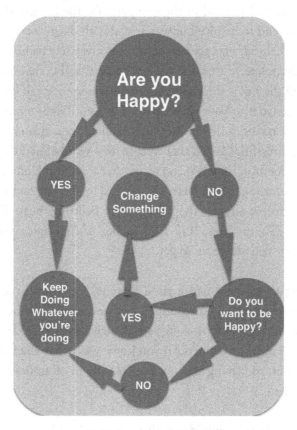

The chart above maps out this very simple formula, yet it is quite challenging to actually implement. It all bottles down to the choices we make and the risks we are willing to take. We can choose to survive miserably by remaining where we are or we can choose to seek happiness by making changes. Changing is not easy because it forces us out of our comfort zone (yes, a miserable survival can still be a comfort zone compared to the Big Unknown). But remaining there means we allow the vicious cycle to continue, and maybe even worsen. Do not wait until it is too late!

At one of my earlier jobs, I used to be seated next to a miserable old gossip who had worked in the company for the longest time. She would pretend to be nice but was armed with daggers ready to stab you from behind. Her greatest talent was creatively padding up her simple job scope so that she seemed more valuable than she really was. And she knew the right people, so trying to speak up against her was suicidal to your own career. I did not like listening to her gossip but trying to ignore her high-pitched incessant chatter was also very stressful. I lasted that torture for a year before I decided to change something and move on to another company. Unfortunately, in trying to break the vicious cycle, I ended up moving on to another world of deeper stress – the world of my belittling boss. After all, as Forrest Gump states, "Life is like a box of chocolates, you never know what you are going to get."

In trying to ensure I had a fixed income, I constantly reminded myself that for things to change I had to change. I thought that things would get better as long as I changed, even the things I had no control over. I felt the devil you knew was better than the devil you did not, so leaving was not the solution to an unhealthy work environment.

In spite of what the public may think, panic disorders and anxieties is not a sign of weakness. It is a condition of trying to remain strong for too long a period of time. In my 13 years of working life, I chose to move four times but within the same industry. During the earlier years, I did not immediately move on. I withstood and embraced every challenge I faced. I was not easily depressed by situations.

I only decided to exit the industry totally after I found that every place I went had the same issues, which were stifling and oppressive. My endurance finally reached its climax on 3 October 2010, the day I realised I had to break free not just from one company but from the environment that seemed to attract the worst in some people.

It is important to identify the cycle that triggers the anxiety and panic attacks, especially the vicious ones. Upon identifying, break it and change the cycle. After all, both the cycle and the future belong to us. It is entirely up to us to keep it or change it. Opportunities come in various forms. Ask yourself what is good for you. What makes you a happier soul? What can you do to help yourself? Write these down on a piece of paper to affirm the facts. Thinking is not enough. Sometimes, we need to write your reflections and look over them to remind ourselves what is most important in life. Few can argue that health should top this list of priorities. Without, health, no amount of wealth can keep you going. Yet, when the situation demands it, without us realising it, health slips down to rock bottom and our focus is channelled more to trading more and more time to just earning an income. We assume our health will remain as it is even without our attention. What a fallacy!

One cycle that keeps me going is the gift of talents that GOD has blessed me with. None of my hidden talents actually took off for huge success during my frustrated years of waiting to exit from the industry I was no longer happy to be a part of, although I never gave up making efforts to knock on the door of opportunity by offering my various creative portfolios for jobs. Nevertheless, it helped me to stay focused and occupied as I constantly produced new videos. With great visualisation and a creative mind as my strongest strengths, I can do anything that uses creativity. For example, cooking, singing, studio photography, filming, video editing, fresh flower arrangement and recently, writing this book to heal and help others in need and search for answers to heal.

I have also produced an album of my song compositions entitled "Solitude". The album comprises 12 songs that are meant to inspire people and break stigmas of mental conditions. The 12 songs are stories of my consistent falls and rises.

Prior to depression and producing an album during the process of my recovery, I had channelled my strengths into gaining various small achievements and I constantly updated my portfolios of artwork online. Even when nothing happened, I kept moving on and creating something new for myself. I constantly attempted to improve myself and did the best I could. I am still dumfounded that the belittling attitude of my last boss could lead me to such long term depression that I forgot for a time that I even had all these strengths and talents. Thankfully, they were just forgotten but not lost forever. With soul searching and the determination to recover, I am picking up the pieces and building myself anew.

Reflection

- As we go through life, we will go through many cycles of opportunities and dangers
- When you are trapped in a vicious cycle (one that keeps you unhappy and makes you sick), you have to decide if it is worth it.
- In a truly oppressive cycle in which you have no control over the environment, it is not enough to say that you should

change yourself in order to be happy. Sometimes breaking away is the only option.

- Moving on is indeed fraught with danger. Nevertheless, if the alternative is paying the price with your health, you should take the risk. God will show you a way out. Just do not lose sight of your strengths.

- Each time we break the vicious cycle and overcome our predicaments, it is a form of rebirth. Your mind needs to be reunited with the rest of your body, especially your heart. Know that you can rise even if you fall.

- You are who you are; the illness is part of you but not the sum of you. Be proud of every move you have made to break a vicious cycle and never look back to a cycle that did not work for you.

!

SEVEN

Love and Hope

Sometimes when life gets too tough to deal with, we tend to forget that love is actually everywhere to assist us in moving forward. A problem seems light and manageable when love acts as a pillar of support. But we need to learn to see, feel, acknowledge and accept the love that is all around us.

When I was unwell, I had so much love offered to me but I failed to see or feel it at that moment. My mind was too bewildered by the physical and mental reactions within me. I have three beautiful and loving siblings. I have a best friend cum housemate who takes excellent care of me. My parents are very supportive and understanding. I have 11 glamorous pussycats and they are the colours of my life. Basically, I was blessed with love surrounding me. However, at the low points of my life when panic attacks were unbearably frequent, the pain clouded my mind and I was judgmental, of myself and others.

Prior to writing this Chapter 7 featuring Love and Hope, I had undergone extreme panic attacks many times a day for many weeks. I was unable to do many things. I could not bring myself to write this chapter as my mind went totally blank. I lost track of time, too exhausted from fighting against the attack. I did whatever I was supposed to do according to my therapy sessions, especially the technique of breathing properly, but all seemed in vain. It was frustrating as my body and mind were in the midst of a catastrophic war. I felt like my world was about to crash anytime because the ordeal was unbearable.

I decided I could no longer write and that my hopes and dreams to help others by getting this book published was not going to happen. I was so vulnerable I began harbouring thoughts of death at the back of my head. However, one part of me remained defiant – I still wanted to survive.

My mother – a bottomless spring of love

I decided to pick up my mobile phone to call my mum, which represents all time LOVE. The moment I heard her voice, I poured all my emotions to her seeking salvation under her wings of love. Her voice has always been the first step to my enlightenment. My mum had gone through so much in life and survived such horrible obstacles that, to a certain extent, she has attained permanent inherent peace. She did not become frantic when she heard my ridiculously panicky voice gasping for breath and hyperventilating hard. Conversely, her calm posture helped me to ease off a layer of the pain almost immediately. That was love in action.

Giving love to receive love

One month earlier, I had a similar violent attack. My mind was on a roller-coaster ride. At the time, my mind was forcing me to look into and deal with not my current problems but to consider minutely possible problems that could arise not just days ahead but weeks and months ahead, all in a flash. It was a race of the mind that put me in a twilight zone of experiencing false evidence regarding all the bad things that could happen to me. Things that I was afraid to undergo. I kept searching high and low for options and solutions where time was crucial. This mind-racing drained my mind so much that I felt like banging my head against the wall and end it. Fortunately, before I could do that, I came across a message from a good animal lover friend by the name of Rosidah, who was in distress herself. She had found three new-born orphaned kittens abandoned in a shoebox. At that time, Singapore was in the midst of the infamous regional haze due to forest clearing in Indonesia. My friend had managed to save the kitties but fretted that she could not foster the new-borns, as she had to work the next day. New-born kittens are very fragile by nature and require feeding every three hours.

Desperate to end the mind racing issue, I immediately volunteered to foster the three orphaned kittens. Even in my desperate phase, I was hopeful that by fostering the kitties and feeding them with milk, I could change the pattern of destructive mind racing. Instead of focusing on fast forward thinking, I made a firm decision to myself to OFFER love and regard the three orphaned cute kittens as my HOPE.

And so I did what I had to do. I took them home and focused on providing them the best care possible.

There was actually one other reason I was so convinced I had to foster these kittens, a pain festering in the deep recesses of my past.

When I was still a small boy, I once came across a box of new-born kitties abandoned in a box on my way home after school. With love and enthusiasm, I placed the box in a safer warmer shelter before returning home. The following day, when I revisited the box, it was filled with ants - all five kitties were dead and decomposing. I remember grabbing the box of dead kittens and frantically running, thinking the kittens could be saved. Only after running aimlessly until my legs could not carry my weight any further, I came to accept that there was nothing else I could do. The sight of the decomposing bodies left me traumatised. The disturbing discovery would continue to haunt me for many years to come.

At 36, out of the blue, the opportunity of overcoming this nightmare of my past appeared just as I was at the brink of despair because of mind-racing. I knew the kittens were a blessing and that I had to go through the fostering program to overcome the tragedy of my past.

My personal principle of dealing with furry friends is that I care for them meticulously. I provide them with a clean home and loads of tender loving care. Some of us may not be fated to have children of our own, but there are always ways to give and receive love. Indulgence in loneliness and self-pity is simply a choice.

The three new-born kittens were just two weeks old when I brought them home. They were super tiny and it was my very first time nursing the new-borns. As they were too young, I had to use a syringe to feed them. I set my alarm clock to three-hour intervals to remind me. It turned out to be exactly the therapy I needed to switch the pattern of my thoughts. Instead of living in an uncontrollable fast-forward future within my mind, I forced myself to live in the present for the sake of my kittens.

My own healing was clearly cat-related. For you it may be different. You will discover a passion that could change your karma of pain, but only when you decide to change it. Week by week, these kittens grew and watching them grow was PEACE. Personalities started to emerge. By the fourth week, genders were more apparent and I named them Chermaine, Lucas and Louisa.

Chermaine is the most observant kitty among them. At that young fragile age, they needed assistance to defecate. Stimulating their genitals allows kittens to defecate naturally. Chermaine would spontaneously lift up both of her hind legs to allow me to stimulate her for defecation!

Lucas was initially weaker than the girls. He regained his strength after I fed him with energy food as prescribed by the vet. By the time they were ready to have their food via bottle, Lucas had become stronger than the girls.

Louisa is fearless. She is as small as my palm but is never intimidated by things bigger than her. She loves sucking and licking my fingers like a lollipop.

I placed their little sanctuary box next to where I slept so that I could monitor these angels. These new-born kitties became mindful of my movements and reacted to my voice. There have been many moments when, fully fed and content, they would huddle together and observe me as I slept. I could feel they were observing and watching me. By the fourth week with me, they did not wake me in the middle of the night for milk and the moment my eyelids opened, the three cuties would literally jump with joy because I was alive and food was on its way. It is indeed amazing how even animals react to LOVE and HOPE.

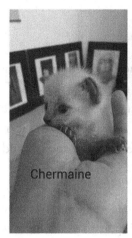
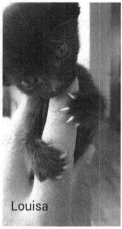
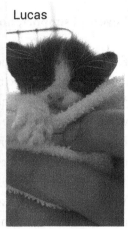

It felt like having three minions from the 'Despicable Me' movie surrounding me. I have learnt that even when circumstances dictate that we do not get recognition from human beings, we can still be appreciated by God's other creations just by being kind to them.

Monty, the dog that saved my life from suicide, gets along well with the three kitties, behaving like an elder brother. Monty gets very excited whenever it is feeding time for the babies.

Personally, I strongly feel that we humans need good relationships, especially between siblings and parents, to be truly happy. Nevertheless, some may just not be blessed with such bonds due to personal reasons and circumstances. If that is the case, my pets are evidence that if we choose to look on the brighter side of life and give ourselves a chance to shower love and hope, somehow, somewhere, we can still enjoy love, at least from other animals.

When my direct family is occupied and unavailable for me, my furry kids have been there to nurse the wounds of my panic struggles.

Love and support, not judge

Family support and understanding is very crucial towards improving one's condition. I use the term "improving" rather than "recovery". Mental conditions require tons of courage and patience. I hate the word recovery because there have been many times in the past when I thought I had recovered. Then I would suffer a relapse and I would fall deep into the dark tunnel again.

Your loved ones want and hope that you can recover soon. But they need to understand that there is no such thing as soon. Rome was not built in a day. Mental conditions need time to improve. No matter how long it takes to recover, for patients encountering panic issues, from my experience, it is better to focus on small steps such as improving your condition. Move on to the next step only when you are ready.

One example is the cassette tape, an example more familiar to people living in the 80s. When on play mode, there are times when our cassette tape would get entangled due to the fast forward and rewind functions. We would slowly remove the cassette tape and if the cassette tape could still be saved, we would use a pencil or pen to gently role the two holes of the cassette to realign the tape. The quality of the recovered sound depended on the severity of the entanglement.

So too with our mental health. There are times when life goes smoothly and I think and feel positive with the help of medication. I am able to function normally and hope surges in my heart. Unfortunately, these feelings of hope often fade and the need to control and persevere is a huge challenge when the antidepressants no longer work on my body. When my mind gets entangled as in the cassette tape, silence, peace and tranquillity is needed to untangle the thoughts.

While the support of my loved ones is appreciated, they cannot urge me to consider my choices quickly; such stress will only worsen my condition. And when I am judged for the choices I make by people do not really understand my condition, it is even worse. When the medication wears out and I am forced to think through things quickly, it feels like my two feet are chained with heavy weights and I am pushed to the sea to drown. It take time and patience to get back on track.

The role of family, trusted friends, soul mates and buddies is to gently help you back on track with support, not to urge the patient to recover quickly.

Reflections

I realise I am blessed with love in three different and precious ways:

- My direct family members and true friends constantly support and lift my spirits when I am in an abyss.
- Choosing to be an animalrescuer has also helped. I understand now that God sent animals to me to show me love even when my loving family are not able to because of their own personal commitments. Sometimes, I am judged because I spend quite a bit to feed my pets but the returns I have received as a result are priceless.
- Last but not least,I have felt the love of God during my travails, in the perfect timing of coincidences. I believe only God knows what will happen in the next step and chapter of my life. I do not know what will happen to me tomorrow but "now" is my responsibility. The least I can

do is to just go with the flow of HIS plans and choose to be a survivor because he keeps giving me reasons to survive. Sometimes – in fact most times – when I request something big from God, it does not come or it does not come easy. Yet, even more amazing are the unexpected gifts from HIM to me. I am constantly amazed by them, so much so that my speculations about the mystery of His gifts itself trigger panic attacks. But then again, I survive thanks to HIM.

EIGHT

Support and Visualisation

For people who suffer from panic conditions, support is the vehicle that carries us forward. The driver of the vehicle of support has ultimately to be you, yourself. It is you alone who can actually ensure that you survive panic and anxiety.

Panic attack is a manifestation of overwhelming fears deep within. My fear of survival after developing a work disability and losing my job escalated many uncertainties and fears within myself. I began to be unable to exit my home and crowd was a huge problem for me. Moving vehicles made me confused. Living in a cosmopolitan city with a high standard of living filled up more blanks in my mind with fears.

When my savings began to dry up, I decided to sell my apartment in order to sustain myself. It was a very tough decision to make as I had invested a lot of emotions, time and money to realise a cosy uncluttered home and loved it very much. Within just a short period of time on the market, my beautiful nest, the place in which I sought sanctuary from the public, was sold. The temporary cash proceeds helped with subsequent home rentals. Rentals were not cheap either. Deposits and moving required money. Eventually that too dried up.

Fortunately, I was given financial support at the time by the very generous people around me but this came with a latent pressure to get well as soon as possible. It seemed to me that there was an urgency to get well in case I lost the shelter I was being offered. Many times I felt that I was a burden and, as a result, I harboured suicidal thoughts.

I know suicide does not solve problems, but when faced with depression, the issue becomes more complex. A healthy mind generally regards suicide as foolish. However, when the mind is bewildered, it is not a thought that we can control easily. Only faith in GOD and Strong Willpower enables us to shut those thoughts out. It is a roller coaster battle where I have to fight myself and affirm to myself daily that giving up means being an irresponsible daddy to my kittens. It would also be unfair to my loving family and my best friends who have supported me so much.

This is when, along with support, visualisation plays a role in helping me stay afloat.

First, I remind myself that I have much that GOD has given me that I have not yet acknowledged. If we keep choosing to focus on the problems, it is hard for solutions to emerge from our minds. Constantly focusing on problems will inevitably lead to self-pity. Self–pity is tiresome as it triggers a vicious cycle of mourning within us. Therefore, with the decision to allow support to penetrate into our minds, we need to allow our minds to be attuned to positivity.

Being positive is a choice. Nobody can tell or force you to be positive. Only you can decide if you want to be positive on the overall outlook of your medical condition. Happiness is all about making the choices in life and what you do with your **right now**.

Not what you did before or in the future. It is **now** that determines the next step of future choices. We have to act upon the choice of wanting to recover each time we fall because we still have the ability within us.

There are two scenarios with regards to persons with mental issues.

Category One: Direct family members are fully supportive towards recovery as caregivers.

Category Two: Family support does not exist.

Do yourself a favour, be honest with yourself. Which category are you in? If you fall under category one, there is no reason for you to give up on yourself because your family and loved ones have not given up on you.

Even if you fall under category two, it is not the end of the world. Avoid self-pity and seek support from organisations that can help you move forward.

I fall under category one, whereby my direct family members - mum, dad, three siblings and a brother-in-law - provide me with unbelievable support and love. They know, understand and acknowledge my strengths and weaknesses. There are also various supporters who do not really know me well but love and support me from a distance.

While I appreciate all their well wishes and prayers, I need to remind myself that their lack of information and understanding can sometimes hinder my recovery process. I receive many well wishes expressing the hope that I will recover 'soon' or 'as soon as possible'. Unfortunately, the word 'soon' somehow automatically sets a deadline in my head to become well which is a pressure in itself. I need to remind myself that that is not what my supporters mean; they only wish the best for me.

For my worst days of severe anxieties and consistent panic attacks, I have drawn up a plan for myself to focus on just four points of reference. By limiting my focal points, I find I am better able to move forward, one step at a time, day after day.

Below is the chart that I personally laid out for myself to kick-start my journey of recovery by visualising four pillars of support.

Four pillars of support I focus on to keep my sanity.

1. Faith in GOD	2. Love from family and friends
3. Therapeutic sessions (Based on individual personal interests)	4. Belief in myself

Pillar 1: Faith

Faith is potent as a lifeline for recovery, be it faith in God or even someone in whom you trust. Keep calm and have faith that you will and you can recover. A strong lifeline to hang on will eventually rebuild your inner strength to move on.

Pillar 2: Love from family and friends

My love language is touch. As much love as I received from my parents and siblings, we never hugged much after reaching adolescence. This was probably because we were too shy and possibly because we never really thought about it. Ever since I became unwell, however, we have started hugging more and it has made a huge difference. Touch instantly connects the other's love directly with my soul and is an affirmation of his or her love, especially when the other is my dad or mum.

Pillar 3: Therapeutic sessions

Besides undergoing professional therapeutic sessions with my case manager, psychologist and psychiatrist, my cats have kept me strong. Prior to my panic conditions and depressions, I was been a responsible worker. When I became ill and unable to exit my home, my depression could have been worse if not for my cats. My principle of being a responsible pet owner – ensuring their daily hygiene and welfare - overcame all other considerations and kept me anchored to the real world.

The benefits? Unconditional tender love from my pets that only animal lovers will understand.

Pillar 4: Belief in oneself

This is probably the toughest pillar among the four pillars to uphold when weighed down by depression or panic. This is because you are alone on this; only you can build this pillar for yourself.

For example, in my case, severe anxiety had reduced my memory capacity and affected my self-esteem. To counter that, I took the initiative to constantly stimulate my brain.

When crowds became too much for me to handle, I refused to stop socialising. Instead, I looked out for group session psychotherapy, which slowly but surely helped me to look and feel normal when facing society. This is important because social participation will be necessary when I step out one day to again earn a living.

Another step I have taken for myself was based on the advice of an 80-year-old elderly friend of mine, Rosie, who passed on a few years back. She reminded me to never stop reading or being mindful of my surroundings if I wanted my brain to last longer. Live every moment, she said. Keep educating my mind. Those were her last words to me. Never would I have imagined that such simple advice would have such a positive impact on my life during my worst days. May she rest in peace.

Believing in myself and having a positive outlook also means forgiving myself for my mistakes.

> **Fear Less, Hope More**
> **Eat Less, Chew More**
> **Whine Less, Breathe More**
> **Hate Less, Love more**
> **And good things will be yours**
> **- Swedish Proverb**

Reflection

- Every one needs support to get through depression and anxiety disorders.

- Look at your situation and decide what your pillars of support are. They could include:

  o Faith in God
  o Family and friends
  o Professional therapy sessions, group therapy sessions and even animal therapy
  o Yourself

- Develop your skills as much as you can on your better days by reading widely and working on your talents. Improving yourself leads to better self- esteem and makes **you** into a formidable pillar for yourself.
- Last but not least,be kind to yourself,and forgive yourself your mistakes, and peace will be within your reach.

Severe Panic Attack

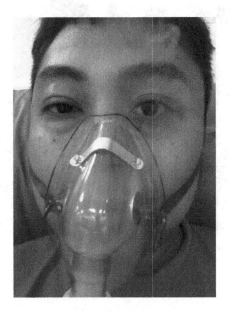

Overcoming Drastic Weight Gain and Loss

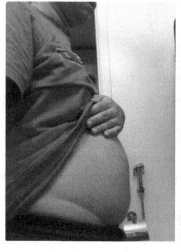

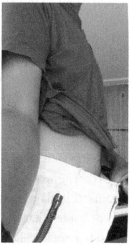

before - 75kg After - 60kg

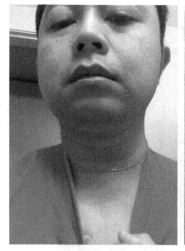

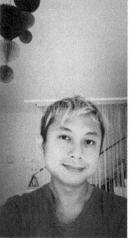

NINE

Relationship, Friendship and Trust

Someone sent me a message through the social media when I shared my condition online. He stated that he felt helpless because he did not have a clue as to how to help me. This is one of the reasons why I decided to write this book.

If you, my dear reader, is suffering from a mental condition yourself, as long as you are not clueless about your condition, and you have a strong desire to recover, there is no need to feel helpless. You need to ensure, of course, that you put into action all your therapy session exercises and that you regularly consume your doctor's prescriptions. You will find a light at the end of the tunnel. And friends can be a valuable part of the journey towards that light.

Similarly, if you are a concerned friend, even if you are not the main caregiver, you can be extremely important in another's road to recovery. It is normal to feel helpless because much is in the hand of the patient himself, and the road to recovery is arduous. The thing to remember is that *speedy* recovery is not what you should wish for your friend with a mental condition. Instead wish him well and support him towards a *steady* recovery.

In this chapter, I will try to explain the expectations of a person with mental issues with regard to their loved ones, and hopefully friends and caregivers will understand how best they can help when a person they care for is assailed by panic or other mental disorders.

True friends are worth their weight in gold

Initially, I used to think that it was wise to expect nothing from anyone else, because friends come and go from your life. Either they get new responsibilities and commitments which prevent them from giving us much of their time, or they may simply find new friends that suit their current needs better.

However, I have realised that some people value being true friends. They will stick by your side during the worst days of your illness. Support from these good friends eventually developed into one of the pillars of my strength.

If you wish to be such a friend, do recognise that such great friendship comes with unconditional commitment. In my case, I understood such friends are rare. So instead of being disappointed or feeling helpless and lonely with the many friends I have, I took the opportunity to filter my friends while I was struggling to survive.

Quality not quantity

Surviving for a day means a lot and takes a lot of courage. Kindness from a friendship is simply an added bonus to my life. As I matured, I avoided any expectations of a shoulder to cry on from friends until I gradually identified those who naturally and sincerely gravitated to my side. These are the truly great friends. During difficult moments, I remind myself I do not need lots of friends to make me feel better. I have programmed myself to believe that I am the most important person I need to make crucial decisions that will make me better or worse. Only then, help from the people who are concerned and who understand my situation will make its way to me. Panic disorder, severe anxieties and depression are complex situations; not everybody can understand and help unless they are equipped with correct information.

Informed friends make the best friends

Without the right information about panic disorder, a well-meaning friend may sometimes feel misunderstood or be misunderstood. Some people choose to keep quiet and remain silent when interacting with a person who has panic disorder because they believe it will help to avoid words that trigger panic attacks. The truth of the matter, however, is that the secret of preventing an attack is to keep a conversation going and listening to the patient consistently. Talking about good things, sweet memories or even moments that invoke laughter provides the needed stimulation to eliminate the panic attack.

Once, I performed singing jazz as the contribution of a recovering patient for World Mental Health Day. Knowing that I am no good with crowds, I stayed in the dressing room while waiting for my performance. During that time, I distracted myself with the stories of the doctors and patients around me with regards to my condition. I was able, by the grace of God, to perform that day without succumbing to an attack.

Stand by my side, don't text me

If you care about someone who suffers from panic attacks, there is one other important thing to remember - face-to- face contact to affirm your love for the patient is invaluable. Living in a cosmopolitan city means earning income becomes the most important priority. Everybody is busy. With technology at your fingertip, people no longer feel the need to come up close and personal in order to communicate. Nevertheless, when one is in a vulnerable and unsteady state of mind, a person needs the real human touch and direct words of affirmation that life can get better.

If not, untimely death could be the result. Mental block is a scary fact of mental illness. Once I accidentally had an overdose despite organising my medication in little boxes because I had a mental block. You can forget days due to a mental block. There was another time I was so depressed with a mental block that I actually cut my own hair, unevenly and unknowingly. My head had to be fully shaved due to the damage once I realised what I had done. Nevertheless, I was lucky I had not accidentally killed myself instead.

Further, certain things normal people take for granted and do unthinkingly can require a lot more effort and time for a person taking drugs to control their mental condition. I lose my coordination sometimes because of what is called the 'serotonin syndrome'. Opening a simple padlock would take me quite a while and I have to battle the tendency to panic as a result. I have lost my house keys many times no matter how well I organise my life. Therefore, having friends around physically to zone us in when we have mental blocks is not just a luxury, it can actually save a life.

Unfortunately, most friendly messages I receive come through my mobile phone. When in depression, fairly or unfairly, I doubt love messages that are based in text. I simply cannot grasp the concept of love through text messages. It is even sadder when people who proclaim they love you in social media, and have lengthy conversations about love and care, have nothing to talk about when you meet them in person. It makes me think that people who do not have mental conditions sometimes live in a more unrealistic world than the one who has the mental illness!

On my part, I constantly express my feelings in writing to distract myself from mental blocks and panic attacks. I also write long text messages to my direct family and trusted friends to share my thoughts and stimulate my mind.

Gravity

Much as I am blessed with various ways to distract my mind, there are times I simply cannot do so. When I cannot, I struggle to overcome my mind racing. Caregivers and concerned friends, if you cannot imagine what this struggle is like, do watch the movie "Gravity". Watch how Sandra Bullock's character struggles to breathe when she is disconnected and lost in space in a space suit. Without gravity, she has to grab anything she can to survive. There are times she feels she can no longer fight because having the willpower to fight to survive is simply not easy. When my mind drifts and when my own mind is against me, it feels like my mind is lost in space and hoping desperately for some gravity; human connection is that gravity which we grab as a lifeline.

Real communications is therefore crucial to support a person with depression and other forms of mental conditions. You may say a hundred or a million times through text messages and social media that you love someone. But if you are not there for the person you claim you love who is fighting mental illness, you are not even close to creating trust inside them that survival is possible. So if you really care, please communicate and care through direct eye contact. My survival is purely based on the ropes of hope reeled out by the people who actually surround me.

Personally, I loathe revealing the chaotic part of my mental illness to my loved ones. I still have the capability of dressing up well and covering my weaknesses with grooming. Strangers will not have a clue that I am struggling to survive. When happy drugs kick into my body, I can remain calm and collected temporarily. I can, at such a time, even allow all input from well-meaning but misinformed people around me – whose advice and gossip could actually cause my condition to deteriorate – to enter through one ear and to come out through the other. But that does not mean my brain does not capture such input. Somehow, it lingers in the brain. Eventually, looking well became a necessity to survive because people did not want to see the ugly truth about me.

During bad days, when the drugs were not working well, I can be impossible. Panic disorder falls under the category of mood disorder too. My mood can swing like a pendulum. One moment I would be a happy soul and the very next moment I could feel like wreck. At such times, all the words people used to describe me, what people will think of me, the possibility that I might lose my loved ones – all the "What Ifs" would assault my mind relentlessly.

At such times, if I had no one to talk to, I would be screaming out aloud. It is not something I can control; my mind is literally disconnected from my body.

At the dressing room, before my performance, I could not stop crying when listening to the stories being exchanged because I realised we shared the same sentiments.

After crying so much, I had to compose myself before I could sing. While I was on stage and singing, I could see the faces of the people who were enjoying my performance. They were on medical drugs just like me to control their own disorders. Suddenly, after the first song, I got emotional because I could feel them. To me, they were fighters. They had been strong for too long overcoming challenges in life. Even when unwell, they were still fighting and rooting for me. The smiles on their faces showed many signs of being a survivor.

My fellow panic order survivors, please understand that it is perfectly normal for you to have friends who genuinely care about you but who do not understand your struggle. If they have never seen you in your panic, or held your hand while you are having difficulty breathing, they simply are incapable of understanding what you go through. There is no point in expecting more from them. On the other hand, a total stranger can become a great friend who understands you just by happening to be present when you fall. God sent me an angel of mercy during one such severe panic attack. I had no one I knew around me and I met her at the hospital itself. She accompanied me into the emergency room and persistently held my hand when I thought I was going to die. She kept assuring me with words of encouragements that I was going to be okay. She is now someone I really respect and has become a true friend. Her name is Penny.

Therefore, besides family, friends who are sincerely concerned and, most importantly, friends who have witnessed your ups and downs with regards to your situation can be invaluable in helping you survive. Do not reject them. If a friend wishes to lend his ear to listen to your problems or offer a shoulder to cry on, be appreciative. Denial of a problem will never solve your problem. Willing friends like these are a blessing and part of your solution.

True friends are not only friends for laughter but also for difficult times when we cry together. Include them in planning ahead as to what can be done for you to become better.

Long-term commitment

But friends who decide to help, please remain for the long haul. It is worse to be a good friend for a while and then leave when the going gets tough, especially if you have gained the trust of someone who suffers from mental disorder. I would go so far as to say that is much worse than not ever showing you care. I have had friends who were initially supportive but decided later that my condition was too much for them to take. They left and decided not to continue talking to me. It is extremely painful when a person who has impacted your life positively and helped you during difficult times abandon you. Fortunately for me, although I was demoralised by such persons, because I was constantly surrounded by those who chose to remain steadfast, I did not collapse despite such abandonment.

Kindness will attract true friends

And I have found that when you try your best to recover and to help others in any way you can, true friends will suddenly appear to lift you up when your family is unable to be there for you.

For example, just by getting involved in animal rescue, I became connected with some great friends. Friends who would always be there when you need them. Friends who are sincere in helping and most importantly, friends who understand your condition deep enough to convert panic into laughter.

I have always been a believer that laughter is the best medicine. Have you ever laughed out so loud that you forget all your troubles? Laughter is always better than crying.

Apparently, I make people laugh simply by laughing. I tear a lot when laughing about something really funny. The messy tears on my face while laughing at the same time have made many of my friends who know me very well want to constantly make me laugh. I suppose my unique laughter outlook is contagious and gets them to laugh and forget their troubles too.

Reflection

If you wish to help a person with mental conditions:

- Take time to understand his condition. Awareness leads to understanding and compassion.
- Take time to be with him physically on a consistent basis, especially when he has an attack. Only then you will gradually understand the struggle, and you may actually be saving a life.
- Advising your friend is not necessary. Instead talk about pleasant things, laughter works miracles.
- Persevere and remain with him for the long term; if you walk out you could do more damage than if you never made friends in the first place.

If you are a person with mental conditions:

- Be aware that a few good friends is better than many uncommitted ones.
- Show your appreciation when you are able to; let them know how you feel.
- Also find ways to help others – great friends will then find you!

TEN

Just do it: Action = Reaction

Nearly giving up

When I decided to write this book, my mind raced far forward and I was afraid to even start. Even after I started writing, there were many times I was afraid to continue because my mind raced towards the editing and publishing processes. I was very afraid of rejections and disappointments. Yet I pushed on. While nobody knew what the future held for me, the least I could do was to put my thoughts into words. It was a long process - there were days when I could write continuously without resting but there were many more days and months where I could not even write a sentence.

After I had written most of the chapters, but not completed the book, I nearly threw in the towel. I was experiencing too many mental blocks due to the side effects of my medication and I was also suffering from stress.

The breakthrough

It was about that time that a charitable organisation supporting mental conditions discovered my singing talent and viewed my website. I was invited for a meeting to discuss a singing performance for one event to break stigmas towards mental conditions. Being cooped up at home most of the time, my anxieties levels were high. I did not know if I could cope with a meeting. I walked to and fro feeling anxious just before the meeting. I became overly paranoid about the way I groomed and what I wore. I have always had a need to hide my anxieties behind my fashion statements. People say when you look good, you feel good. I believe that and grooming is important to me when I need to meet anyone.

Eventually, I composed myself and managed to meet the president of Club HEAL, Dr Radiah Salim. Club HEAL is an organisation in Singapore to assist and empower persons with mental illness to regain confidence in themselves and others in their journey towards community reintegration. I went for the meeting and everything turned out just fine.

By deciding to change the way I thought in a positive way, I made a small difference in my life which in time became more manageable as I took one opportunity and step at a time.

I had so many insecurities about my strengths, financials and future but, somehow, that has changed ever since I started to socialise more with recovering patients and people who had faced other forms of disorders and who could understand me deeper for a start.

Developing the skill of zoning out

By nature, I have always been bothered about what other people might say. One opinion can sometimes bother me so much that I fail to move on or do what I feel is right. Sometimes people advise me to follow my heart. And, most times, I do so despite being bothered by opinions. Good and positive opinions were always helpful in guiding my decisions on whatever I intended to do. However, when it came to negative opinions, it took some time for me to develop the skill of zoning out the negative vibes. Just like the saying "Forgiven but not forgotten".

In my case, the ultimate example of words that took too long to get out of my head were the belittling words my final boss used to say to me. Only with time did I realise that such negative opinions and comments were not worth hanging onto.

Now, whenever I have feelings of rage beyond my ability to eliminate, I deliberately choose to focus on doing activities that make me happy. It is just amazing how quickly even the most persistent of negative comments can actually disappear when you master the skill of determining what your *positive* consequent step will be as soon as such thoughts start to linger in your mind.

It is important also to understand that we do not know the reasons people make the negative opinions that affect us so badly. It is likely that these people also have problems, concerns and personal insecurities within themselves, especially underlying issues which have not been resolved. Therefore, seeing someone else possessing certain qualities triggers opinions that may affect your confidence.

When I had to take two months of unpaid leave due to depression, I still had my job. It was a downgrading of sorts; I had lighter duties and a much lower income. Despite that, I still looked upon the brighter side, which was to count my blessings. The possibility that I would feel normal again in two months was a blessing in itself. And having a job, albeit in a demoted position, was still a blessing because it meant I would have the means to pay my mortgage.

My mistake was I failed to remember that people do not change overnight. They need to overcome obstacles similar to mine before they would be able to understand my condition.

Breaking a vicious cycle through action

You can break a vicious cycle when you want it and not just *if* you want it. I did that. I decided to leave my fate to GOD instead of worrying about how I would survive without a job. No one should control your life but yourself. No one can help you but yourself, apart from God. Ironically, when you submit yourself wholly to Him and do what you need to do, other people who love and care for you will be able to help you on your road to recovery.

Personally, I strongly believe that God tests us in life because He loves us. What is life without obstacles? When everything in life is perfectly fine all the time, the soul will be starved. Only by overcoming obstacles, facing problems and making mistakes – yes, that one is a must – do we learn anything of value. If you are a bad cook, you can either choose not to cook ever again when you burn your first toast, or you can continue learning from mistakes until you become a master chef.

The same goes for panic conditions. Today, I regard my panic conditions as a blessing even though I do not enjoy daily panic attacks. My life changed because of them. Yes, I cannot do certain things in life that I used to enjoy, like having great conversations with my ex- colleagues during lunch time. Even though the demands of my job and the working environment were unhealthy, my ex-colleagues and I mostly knew how to control the situation. We worked well as a team for survival.

But, things did not all go downhill because of unemployment. I have gained a lot from the experience. In short, it has been okay not to be okay because I chose to learn from my many mistakes, especially regarding my options on managing my finance to survive unemployment. Just as in the alphabet there are letters A to Z, there are options A to Z. The first idea we consider as a future undertaking is obviously Plan A. But to be safe, we prepare Plan B just in case Plan A does not work. We are even safer if we have a Plan C. When my mind races, my mind cannot control how many plans I make, it strives to attend to one contingency then another – from A to Z. My mind spins like a washing machine as I have too many ideas in my head too fast.

But the same qualities protect me from the procrastinating behaviour of many normal people who, as a result, miss great opportunities or fall into deep trouble. In my case, I have found that this ability is like a gift of premonition from GOD – if I ignore a particular possibility it tends to happen and that leads me to panicky situations.

The other thing that I have come to realise on hindsight is that I had spent most of my life taking action for the benefit of others so much so that I had forgotten that I had a life too. That was a grave mistake but I have learnt from it.

You have every right (and even a duty you owe yourself) to control and manage your stress before it becomes your worst enemy. Seeking treatment early means the possibility of detecting underlying issues early. Early detection provides you with an easier recovery.

For me, it took me three years before I could even bring myself to take the first step towards solving the mystery of my anxiety. For most of those three years, I was afraid. I was fearful of getting out of my home. I was terrified of being misunderstood. I was petrified of going out to work. What if I again had to go under an obnoxious egocentric boss who would irreparably damage my self-esteem? How much was I worth? How much could I contribute to the company? Would I face discrimination again simply because I was single and be expected to spend long hours in the office even though my work for the day was done? Even the sound of the traffic in the central business district triggered panic in me.

I kept questioning how one person's crass insensitivity could lead me to such a nerve-wrecking condition. It was not like I had never faced stress before. I felt that I had managed just as much stress or more for 13 years working, so why now? These questions lingered in my head leading to insomnia and eventually depression.

Now I believe that I could have avoided much of that suffering if I had more information and had received medical treatment immediately. I had never cried to sleep so much in my life.

Unemployment led to more stress when I started losing my savings. I sold my home and rented new premises. Unfortunately those savings dried up faster than I could replace them, and, naturally, my anxiety heightened. Yet, every decision I made regarding rentals had revolved around grabbing opportunities at the right place and the right time. If not for my 'plan fast and take action even faster' personality, I would have lost my savings even more quickly. One fact was evident: despite all the depression and anxieties, when it came to survival, I was still able to plan and execute.

Enjoy your victories, one step at a time

Through therapy, I began to realise the importance of planning for now instead of the distant future. I learnt to anchor small achievements instead of moving on and on and on as soon as I reached a particular milestone. I had omitted to enjoy the accomplishments I had achieved. Therefore, naturally when I worked under someone who had high expectations regarding working hours without paying extra and yet questioned my self-worth, my tolerance climaxed and the resulting emotional avalanche crushed me like a cockroach. Pinned, I was not able to get up for the longest time.

Back to school and acing it

But now, all that is no longer important to me because the fact is I did get up each time I fell. I remember the initial stage of me trying to anchor my achievements. It was not easy. After losing my job, to avoid feeling restless after recovering somewhat but still unstable, my best friend suggested that I go for a short basic filming course to stimulate my mind. Creativity is part of my strengths. And so, I went for a short course at a local institute and started making younger friends. The short course was uplifting for me. From being totally afraid of going out, I pushed myself out of my comfort zone.

It was a very short one-month course but, as usual, I was always serious when it came to assignments. We were required to create a five-minute music video or less as a submission for the short course. The moment I acknowledged an assignment was required, I visualised the end product of what I would like to do even before anyone could even begin to imagine it. I pictured it in my mind. I planned, then executed the plan with a group of young people. It was a Bollywood music video of my own style. The music video turned out exactly as I had visualised in my head and was a roaring success.

That made me a little more confident about myself going out and socialising again. However, I still try to avoid crowded places and busy roads as much as I can, as they confuse me and trigger anxieties.

One day, I packed my bags of cameras and start filming another visualisation of mine for a local music video competition. I did so by myself. I thought why not? Just do it. I had no expectations of winning. All I focused on was achieving the objective of the music video requirement, which was "Dreams and Love and featuring local flavour". I filmed random shots of any type of love that I saw on the streets, which also reflected hope and dreams. I wrote a song, recorded the vocals (which I sang myself), and did my own video editing. Bam! I was the first runner-up for the competition. I won a $3000 cash prize and I spent it all on more filming gadgets since I also won a scholarship to further my studies in Diploma of Filming Production.

When the school administrator broke the news to me, I went to somewhere quiet and had a long cry to myself. Joy beyond my wildest imagination. I could not believe that I had moved on from an environment where I felt stupid and worthless to a brand new situation where there were people who could actually see and appreciate my strengths.

Thinking that my hope for recovery was working well and I could be myself again, I moved one step forward and began to further my education. It meant a lot to me because filming was something I enjoyed doing and my lack of qualifications hindered my progress.

I never really understood the importance of education until I was 35. In my previous corporate career, the higher the education, the bigger seemed the stress. I had seen fresh graduates joining us like fresh blooming flowers all ready to pursue their chosen paths. Their faces were filled with hopes and aspirations. It was simply a matter of time before they withered like dehydrated flowers, pressed and compressed with dead weight after dead weight of unreasonable expectation. Those who learnt the art of pushing responsibilities in the most diplomatic way were the ones who survived.

I felt choked when I witnessed pretentious big fishes pushing responsibilities. No matter how superior they were in the management level and in their capability to make others suffer silently, I also felt sorry for them because, for me, the worst nightmare in life is achieving material things in life but losing the respect and love of those around you.

And so, when I started filming school in 2012, I was all ready to start my life anew. I made huge efforts to hide my anxieties so that no one could see that I had them. It was an experience of a lifetime for me, being 35 and befriending young local and international filming students.

The sudden fall

Unfortunately, at the peak of my excitement and enjoyment of school, I had a sudden relapse that brought me back down rock bottom. I was hospitalised for about three weeks in a mental institution as I went through a phase of psychosis. After only one semester, I could not proceed further with my filming education. It was very difficult for me to bite the bullet. But with time, I did manage to overcome that loss. I managed to direct one short film for the first semester. My principal advised me to keep doing videos and update my portfolio. One fine day, I will achieve my dreams. Everyone who survived that filming course eventually got their paper qualifications but I kept my mind occupied with creating and producing videos. I also made the effort to rescue more animals in need.

Picking myself up again

Time after time, life experiences have taught me one unalterable truth. Life has no remote control for you to change channels while sitting on the couch. I simply have to get up and change directions myself whenever necessary. New ideas may face rejection. Accepting, acknowledging and dealing with disappointment was extremely challenging, but with willpower and big dreams, I have kept the momentum of producing new videos, my vocal recordings and writing.

In one session with my psychiatrist, he suggested that I read or watch the life story of Steve Jobs, the man behind Apple Computers, the IPod, the IPhone, etc. I followed his advice and watched the biographic movie of his life story entitled JOBS. I realised that Steve Jobs and I shared the same ability called visualisation. There are many things I knew I could achieve if I chose not to give up my belief in my visualisations.

When I share my visions, often my ideas are regarded as time bombs that ought to be diffused. I become confused then because my strong visualisation about the possibilities that I can achieve is so strong.

I learnt that being fearless about my own strengths was key. No matter what you dream of, you can do it, with perseverance.

Reflections

- Plan and take action if you wish to change your life. No one can do it but yourself.
- There will always be naysayers who will in stildoubt in you and rejections and disappointments will also pull you down, but be determined to get up again with the belief that God cares and will help you.
- Somehow, someday, if you persevere, somebody will approach you and believe in your vision. Be confident and believe in your strengths yourself.
- If we want to be great we have to take risks and be prepared to lose everything. Start with small things and savour each achievement.

- At the end of the day, make it simple to last your whole life long.
- And remember, regret is the one certain thing if you do not pursue any dream that you envision.

ELEVEN

Counting Blessings Not Misfortune

Regardless of one's religious affinities, anyone who has gone through and risen from misfortunes will somehow learn to understand blessings from a different perspective. Not only is there a reason for everything that happens, everything is also temporary. Good or bad, whatever crops up will sooner or later go away, be it after a short period of time or a longer period of time. In the end, it is just a matter of TIME.

As I have said before, I strongly believe that GOD tests us because HE loves us. Just like parents. They discipline us because they love us and want the best for us. But sometimes, especially during adolescence when we start developing minds of our own, we tend to not agree with certain things that are best for us. Some will heed their parents' good advice while others will be defiant and rebel.

Counting blessings is not something that is easy to do without practice and it is also something that is personal. You need to develop an inner peace deep within yourself where no one can see, feel or intervene but yourself. It is a place that links the conscious mind to the heart.

I remind myself that the past is the past but the present leads to my future. The dark tunnel I have emerged from provides me with the opportunity to experience a new life, even if the light at the end of the tunnel is coloured with panic disorder.

If not for all the pain I had to go through, I would not be the person I am today. I would have remained in the corporate world, stuck in a rut, doing the same things I did over and over again, and hating it.

In general, blessings make our day. Even the smallest pinch of happiness can expand and explode in our heart, filling it with contentment. Some blessings come in disguise and it takes faith and time before you can see it for what it is.

When I had to face my own predicament, I chose to believe that it was a blessing in disguise. It was not easy but it was necessary. During my first year without a job, receiving a scholarship and the thought of continuing my education built baby hopes that things were going to get better. I kept telling myself to believe in my strengths and not dwell on my weaknesses.

The scholarship for filming education was a major blessing, although short-lived. After winning the music video competition and attending school, I had felt rejuvenated. My young and vibrant classmates did not have a clue that I had such an incapacitating illness. I hid my illness well. Whenever I had a mild panic or anxiety attack, I would disappear to somewhere quiet to compose myself again. It was a nice feeling socialising with youths. Their perspective and mine differed, certainly, due to the discrepancy in our ages and our experiences. I was at least 20 years older than those students. Nevertheless, it gave me the opportunity to learn how generation Y, our next generation pool of creative leaders, think.

Twenty-two years ago when I was in high school, I never really enjoyed schooling. I was popular in school based on my various leadership roles and activities with the school band and other performing activities. But, I frequently felt sad, afraid and lonely. I was teased and called names. During those years, peer pressure was quite challenging to deal with. I was not a sportsman like the other boys, but felt that playing football was a totally necessary criterion to be a man and earn respect. I was terrified of physical education sessions as everyone was expected to play some kind of sports after exercising. We started with warm ups and runs followed by the sport of our choice. The boys played either football or basketball whilst the girls played volleyball or badminton. And I was neither here nor there. I had butter fingers and moving balls confused me.

The girls were more tolerant about my weakness and invited me to join them in badminton. Even so, I was never good with games.

Looking back at the various symptoms of panic attacks, I realise that I actually had anxiety problems even during my school days. Unfortunately, they were never diagnosed or dealt with adequately. With the passing of years, these unattended anxieties escalated into raging fires of uncontrollable panic.

This is why my advice to anyone who has overwhelming unattended fears is: please talk to professionals and solve these issues quickly, before they haunt you day and night. Panic attack is a manifestation of uncontrolled fear. The only way to avoid it is to overcome your fears as much as you can.

I have noted earlier that I remind myself frequently that my past belongs in the past and should not mar my future. However, be prepared to face that past - professional therapeutic treatments will always temporarily lead you to your past so that you can solve any unattended business. This will enable you to move on towards your future.

Hospitalisation – a blessing?

Hospitalisation in a mental hospital for treatment was an experience I could never forget in my life ever. My condition was controlled in the ward by medical professionals. Drugs prevented my mind from racing forward, fast and furious. There were sessions of group psychotherapy where the discussions helped make me understand that I was not alone. I also went through mental stimulation exercises conducted by a psychologist. My first hospitalisation was devastating for me. I felt that my future was doomed. Who would want to employ me when I had the stigma of mental illness? How was I to face anyone when I had been so branded? I did not want to accept the fact that the hospitalisation was necessary to stabilise my condition.

But again, I made the decision to trust God - even though it was difficult to BELIEVE in counting your blessings and not your misfortunes, I forced myself to believe that somehow something good would eventually emerge from the episode, if not immediately, then slowly but surely.

As I progressed searching for means and ways to recover, I learnt that, in life, balance was vital. With the right positive mentality, you can overcome anything as long as you are mindful of what is happening to you and break the cycle before it becomes a vicious one.

Each time I decided to count a blessing, and appreciate and enjoy it, I was one small step towards creating a positive mindset for myself.

Second wave attack – a blessing?

The moral of the second wave attack that I experienced was to expect the unexpected. I gave my misfortune some time to go away so that my blessings in disguise could make its way back into my life. There are valuable lessons to be learnt through catastrophes. By being able to move on, in itself, your life becomes richer with knowledge that you have what it takes to survive.

As much as we sometimes feel lost in the storm, there is wisdom in remembering that there are others who are feeling even worse than us. This fact can only be embraced when you have accepted your difficulties and start listening to stories of people who have gone through even more than yourself.

Thanks to technology, with one click, you can many get things done. One example is bill payment. Internet banking saves you a trip to the post office to pay your bills. Even without such technology, with just one click from GOD, our hearts can simply stop beating and we become history. Being given an opportunity to breathe and be alive is itself an unquantifiable blessing - I have understood this fact of life only after I struggled to get better.

Along with the process of recovery, I have also learnt the importance of being thankful for the past, present and future. Every breath we take is an opportunity for us to grow and expand our mind. Without such experiences, we would be very shallow in our thinking. When I was forced to leave the corporate world, the doors to many new experiences opened themselves for me.

My neighour's son

For example, there was a time when I had difficulty understanding and making friends with children. I did not think they were worth having conversations with. When I was stuck at home unemployed, I discovered just how wrong I was.

Every morning, the moment I woke up and after my prayers, I would feed my furry kids – nine cats and three dogs - before I had my own breakfast and medications. I would vacuum and mop the floor, wash the dishes, water the plants, feed the fishes and do the laundry. Then I would be in the porch of my newly rented semi-detached home hanging out the clothes to dry, sweeping the porch area and doing my gardening therapy while the dogs played.

A neighbour's son became excited by the sight of my three dogs and would greet me enthusiastically with comments and questions whenever I was in the porch. Because of my depression, until the drugs kicked in, I would experience a kind of uncontrollable irritation of anything that interfered with my sanctuary and comfort zone. The presence of my neighbour's child, Kim Yong (not his real name), did exactly this as he spoke loudly and got on my nerves. I tried to discourage him by remaining aloof and not maintaining eye contact as he chattered. The fact is, at that time, I did not like speaking to most human beings as I felt that even close friends and relatives had disappointed me.

Nevertheless, because the boy was unstoppable, one fine morning, I finally broke the ice with the irritating pest. I asked him why was he not in school. He put his head down with sadness and shared with me that he was having a year's break from school and was bored to death. I asked why and he responded that he was waiting for school transfers.

Kim Yong shared with me some of his problems and I realised that he expressed himself very eloquently. Even more revealing, he was going through a lot of problems which, if unattended, could lead to possible depression and mental illness in the future. I was astounded. My goodness! Such a young boy and yet facing adult problems? My heart bled for him.

Kim Yong was in love with Laura, an abandoned golden retriever dog that I had rescued. She had been in a bad state of health, with ear infections, when I first met her. She was a female dog that had been used by breeders to breed and sell pups. I suppose when Laura got older and was not able to produce beautiful puppies for the breeder, she was eventually abandoned. Another sad fact of God's creature being exploited. Kim Yong was appalled by the notion of such cruelty. In time, Laura became not only my positive distraction from panic attacks, but also a therapy for the lonely boy.

Reflections

- There are blessings even in suffering, although it will take great discipline and determination to understand them. Trusting in God's great love and looking for the wisdom in his hidden plans always helps.
- Counting your blessings rather than enumerating your problems make blessings more evident.
- There is always someone out there who has suffered more than you. Look out for them and you will be more aware of your own blessings and you will grow into a more empathetic person at the same time.
- It might be easier to give up when faced with extreme anxieties and the horrible turmoil of mind racing, but if you choose to understand and enjoy the process of recovery, every small goal achieved becomes priceless.
- While only patients can actually know how it feels, caregivers should continuously believe in and focus on the strengths of the patient. If you can raise their self-esteem with words of encouragement and touches of love, your support becomes invaluable.

TWELVE

Anchoring Achievements

Patience is a virtue. There were many times when I was over-critical about my circumstances and worried excessively about the future. For the first two years of unemployment, it was relatively easy to be patient and reaffirm to myself that life would get better. However, during my third year of unemployment, I became much more vulnerable.

I was relying at the time 100% on my best friend, Charles (now considered a member of my family) for both a roof over my head and for the expenditures to sustain life. The fear that I might lose my pets led to daily unbearable panic attacks. The world was crashing down on me.

I had difficulty anchoring achievements as I was a perfectionist. Now I tell myself that perfection is boring and prefer to use to term "constipated" to laugh at myself when I worry about perfection.

Anchoring small achievements is important because it leads to bigger achievements. Anchoring and enjoying small achievements is a skill every panic disorder patients must attempt to master over time with practice. It is not easy. However, by talking to someone you are comfortable with or even your psychologist, you will learn to appreciate the anchoring process.

Patients with panic conditions need patience more urgently than ordinary people. We need it to develop in ourselves the higher level of appreciation that makes it easier to confront every trouble that could trigger panic in us. Everyone is capable of patience. We have to find it in us and, upon finding it, it is even more important to learn to hold on to it. Never let go of the patience that we have been blessed with.

There were many days and nights when I cried to myself wondering if I might ever lose my patience in fighting the battle of panic every single day. I knew that losing patience meant losing also the strings of hope that I had weaved within myself to survive.

This was not because I was not counting my blessings. I was fully aware that I had managed to accomplish quite a few things despite my condition, for example winning the music video award and receiving a scholarship to study filming. Also, I was deeply aware that I had a great blessing in the form of my caregivers; my family and friends have been solid pillars of strengths.

But I had to be careful not to compare apples with oranges, and compare myself with persons who achieved other great or greater things. I needed to remind myself that I needed massive courage just to do little things, so achieving even a relatively big thing should be considered even more massive to me. Till now, I cannot imagine how I managed everything that I have achieved. But I have.

Nevertheless, having strengths does not mean they will last forever, especially if we fail to anchor achievements adequately.

To me, anchoring achievements is about pausing and enjoying the moment of NOW and not dwelling on YESTERDAY or worrying about TOMORROW. For one who suffers from panic disorders, it is not just the traumas of the past that may cause trouble for the future. Worrying about tomorrow can affect my life of today. My tomorrows are often fast forwarded to months and, if not controlled by positive distractions, I could easily leap years ahead to things that might or might not happen in the future.

One example is the fear of losing my mum when she passes on. Despite so many obstacles and challenges, my mum has always remained calm when I get too difficult. There were many days when I vented my many frustrations, rage and anger on her. And there are many days when I speak to her via video chat or phone with so much hope, respect, laughter and love. My mum has great poise when dealing with me when I am unwell, with my mood swinging like a pendulum. A man who has nightmares daily will certainly be in pain. For me, my nightmares occur in broad daylight. I cannot imagine being without my mum. How will I survive? This terror haunts me.

However, when I choose to anchor my achievements, I know deep down that there is a possibility of good things happening with or without my mum, which means I will be able to survive. Nevertheless, the fear constantly lingers in my head.

To successfully fight anxiety and its attendant disorders, including panic, agoraphobia, depression and at one point of my life, a Serotonin Syndrome, I need constant motivation.

Besides my mum, my motivation comes in many other forms. My animal rescue missions comprise one huge mountain of HOPE that I can rely on, but rescued animals come with huge responsibilities and being unemployed and financially supported by my family and my caregiver, Charles (who gave a shelter, space and time for me to recuperate with my furry kids) in itself causes insecurities even as it provides comfort. Again, it is about another layer of fear. Fear of losing tomorrow what I have NOW.

Throughout my journey to be well, I have learnt to filter out people who claim they love me but never call to say Hi to me. It does not cost an arm or a leg to call. To me, love is a strong word. I do not believe love is sincere unless proven with action. With my mental condition, I feel betrayed by that word.

Despite knowing my willpower to fight, sometimes people are insensitive of the effort behind those small successes that I have achieved. I then have problems patting myself on the back for my hard work and effort in making my life better. On the other hand, some words of encouragement from the people who say they love and pray for me make a huge difference to me when I try to anchor my achievements.

For example, once on 4 November 2013, I was ranked Number 1 on the charts for the Jazz and Ballad category representing Singapore on an online music channel.

My direct family, some fans and a bunch of people around the world sent me words of encouragements and congratulations. Sadly, some others, whose claims of love I had truly believed in, did not bother to even acknowledge the achievement. Silent treatment is the last thing I needed on my journey of recovery, especially when it comes to anchoring achievements.

Initially, instead of jumping with joy or celebrating a particular achievement, as a result of such response, I would fall into depression again. It took so much effort to gain confidence but only a small disappointment to shut my body down. I then had to withstand days of nausea, migraine and diarrhoea while rebuilding my courage.

To move on, from thereon, I concluded that such people did not really understand the meaning of love. Surviving that, I realised that constant motivation and words of encouragement play a critical role in recovery.

With that outlook, I have chosen now to create an image for myself that people will approve. Therefore, on social media or when meeting people in person, I groom myself, dress up and avoid looking unwell because first impressions count. To me, looking well is important. But to look well, I have to energise myself in solitude. It came to a point where I had to put on a role-play in order to put up singing gigs or when I had to attend any important event of my life.

However, there are times where I choose to be myself. As unwell as I am, I need to accept who I am. The fact is it is tiresome to always worry about what others think of me.

A good friend once reminded me that I did not need many people to understand me. All I needed was one. And I have been lucky to have more than one.

I also underwent several psychotherapies to help me identify the vital signs that trigger my daily panic attacks despite having achieved certain successes throughout my recovery journey. It has been a long and winding road for me.

I have been surprised to discover that while every day may not be good, there is invariably something good in every day when we choose to the see the goodness of every single day.

Instead of going with the flow, I have created the flow of my life. After all, the choice is mine. The past is over and, in my case, I have set my mind to focus more on the state of the moment of now and the future.

I officially launched my debut full album entitled "Solitude" on 15 November 2014, after surviving phenomenal mental health challenges. The album is dedicated to all people around the world facing and battling mental conditions. The completion of my album is probably the biggest achievement I have had to practice anchoring and accepting. There were too many times I wanted to give up but with the support of Club HEAL, the Institute of Mental Health and donations from friends and family, the album was eventually completed and launched.

The "Pop Progressive" CD album genre comprises of 12 songs that I composed and performed sharing my recovery journey. I hope the positive and motivating songs I sing in the album will inspire everyone, regardless of whether they suffer mental conditions or not, to believe that dreams can come true. All we need to do is pour effort from our heart, mind and soul into the DREAM.

The objective of the album is purely to create awareness, break mental stigmas and encourage people with mental conditions to continue believing that life can get better. I wish one day, I could travel around the world meeting survivors as a motivational speaker or singer helping people feel at least better if not great. Personally, the priceless gift to me for readers of this book and listeners to my "Solitude" music album will be knowing that someone out there, anywhere in the world, with mental conditions, now has a better quality of life. I want them to achieve their small and big dreams, earn income confidently, be accepted by society and attain happiness.

Reflections

- In conclusion, as a human being, the most valuable and priceless lesson I have learnt from surviving a panic disorder is that, in order for me to appreciate and be thankful for this wonderful opportunity called LIFE, I have choices:

    o To be in control of my life, to make mistakes, to try new things even if I stumble and fall.
    o By falling, sometimes I get hurt but I can choose to rise again, I can choose to learn more and I can choose to keep growing and expanding my mind.

- The mind is like a gate. I can choose to open my gate:

    o To accept facts, control my emotions and allow great opportunities to enter.
    o I can open it as narrow or and as wide as I wish it to be. The decision is mine.

- There is no doubt that life is like the waves of the sea. There will be times when a storm could bring the waters to a chaotic high and then crash down.
- By controlling the gate of my mind, I can stabilise and transform tsunami waves to that of a calm sea. Even a calm sea has waves. The difference is that calm sea waves are far more manageable to deal with compared to huge waves. The highs and lows are not so far apart, so it is easier to rise up to the highs again when the low starts to take over a situation.

I hope that this book has been helpful to patients or caregivers to move forward with their battles. It is my heartfelt wish that recovering patients will have a beautiful journey and success towards recovery. Remember, you are not alone. And more importantly, do remember that you are a winner each time you choose to have the willpower to survive.

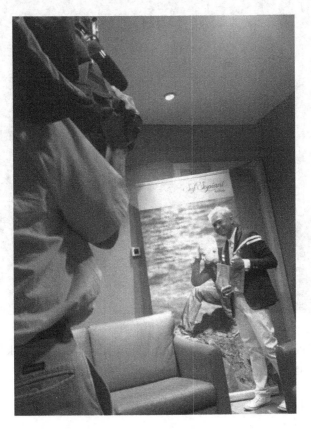

Album Launch for Mental Health Awareness and to Debunk Mental Stigmas

Every little success doesn't come overnight. Successes with pain feels enlightenment with personal satisfactions. Thus, to enjoy the process is key to remain strong if not stronger.

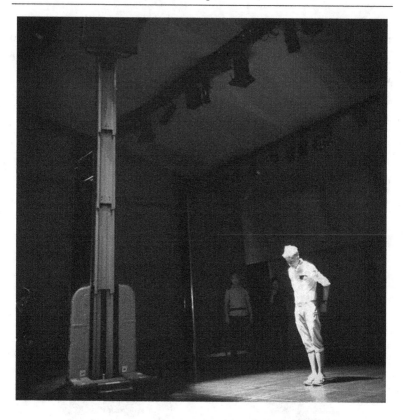

My music artwork concept album is available from the link below.
https://itunes.apple.com/us/album/solitude/id946516691

END